Public Health and Primary Care
Partners in population health

Alison Hill
Director, NHS Supporting Public Health, Oxford, UK

Siân Griffiths
Professor and Director of School of Public Health,
The Chinese University of Hong Kong, Hong Kong

Stephen Gillam
General Practitioner, Luton;

Director, Public Health Teaching, School of Clinical Medicine,
University of Cambridge, UK;

Visiting Professor, University of Bedfordshire, UK

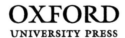

OXFORD
UNIVERSITY PRESS

OXFORD
UNIVERSITY PRESS

Great Clarendon Street, Oxford OX2 6DP

Oxford University Press is a department of the University of Oxford.
It furthers the University's objective of excellence in research, scholarship,
and education by publishing worldwide in

Oxford New York

Auckland Cape Town Dar es Salaam Hong Kong Karachi
Kuala Lumpur Madrid Melbourne Mexico City Nairobi
New Delhi Shanghai Taipei Toronto

With offices in

Argentina Austria Brazil Chile Czech Republic France Greece
Guatemala Hungary Italy Japan Poland Portugal Singapore
South Korea Switzerland Thailand Turkey Ukraine Vietnam

Oxford is a registered trade mark of Oxford University Press
in the UK and in certain other countries

Published in the United States
by Oxford University Press Inc., New York

British Library Cataloguing in Publication Data

Data available

Library of Congress Cataloging-in-Publication Data

Hill, Alison P.
 Public health and primary care / Alison Hill, Siân Griffiths, Stephen Gillam.
   p. ; cm.
 Includes bibliographical references.
 ISBN 978-0-19-850853-3 (alk. paper)
1. Public health. 2. Primary care (Medicine) I. Griffiths, Siân, 1952- II. Gillam, Stephen. III. Title.
 [DNLM: 1. Public Health. 2. Health Care Reform. 3. Primary Health Care. WA 100 .H645p 2007]
 RA425.H45 2007
 362.1--dc22

                                                                        2007003248

Typeset by Cepha Imaging Pvt. Ltd., Bangalore, India
Printed in Great Britain
on acid-free paper by
Biddles Ltd., King's Lynn, Norfolk.

ISBN 978-0-19-850853-3

10 9 8 7 6 5 4 3 2

Whilst every effort has been made to ensure that the contents of this book are as complete,
accurate and up-to-date as possible at the date of writing, Oxford University Press is not
able to give any guarantee or assurance that such is the case. Readers are urged to take
appropriately qualified medical advice in all cases. The information in this book is
intended to be useful to the general reader, but should not be used as a means of
self-diagnosis or for the prescription of medication.

Foreword

It gives me pleasure to write a foreword for a book so very much of its time. The fact that all three authors have been my colleagues gives me added pleasure as I have first hand experience of their huge knowledge and commitment. The public's health in all its many facets has never been so central to Department of Health policy, with its ambition to put people more in control of their own health and health care, to enable and support promoting health, independence and well-being, together with rapid and convenient access to high quality, cost effective services.

The evidence referred to in the ensuing chapters is that a primary care focus is the optimal way to ensure that this ambition is realized. The recent White Papers propose ways of delivering the WHO vision of health and implementing these to provide a holistic approach to primary care—an opportunity indeed. This book with its welcome focus on philosophy, theory and practice gives us the tools to deliver. Any good book should fuel debate, and this book does not disappoint.

The UK general practice registered list of patients is a unique feature even amongst other first contact health care systems. It enables better management of patients who live with long-term conditions, and the new GP contract has created incentives for even better care. The list is, of course, the basis of resource allocation in practice-based commissioning and is potentially a register of the local public health population. That latter potential still needs to be fully realized, but currently there are excellent examples of practice-based public health involvement within the NHS. Another particular feature of primary care which offers continuity is the public health potential of the individual consultation. This applies as much to community nurses, pharmacists and dentists as to doctors, all of whom provide popular and effective care. So primary care sits at that interface between the bio-clinical world, which for chronic illness delivers up to 40 per cent of health gain, and the wider public health approach to the health of the population. This approach may contain paradoxes and lead at times to local tensions, but no other organizations can potentially deliver so much. The authors well describe the essential support required.

We need to combine the new public management with what is described as the new public health management. Failure to deliver targets that benefit the public and failure to keep to budget cannot be good management of the public's monies. Access to primary care is of value to those who live in areas of socio-economic need. Julian Tudor Hart's inverse care law needs to be properly addressed in primary care. Access to services such as Walk-in Centres aids that process, and their size and scope pose no threat to an active traditional primary care that itself needs to expand. There are plenty of incentives to do so.

But what about the money? I describe rationing as the delay to or denial of appropriate and effective care. Yet much of what we traditionally provide is neither. I cite as an example the 20 per cent of hospital budgets spent on that outmoded concept known as out-patients. When we also review the lack of evidence of many clinical interventions, the monies add up. There is also a public health imperative to protect people from unnecessary interventions. We have generally failed to address such cost ineffective activity. Practice-based commissioning, being clinically led, offers our best option. The generalist has never had such potential for a better future.

A reinvigorated public health is essential to support primary care to fulfil its potential further while retaining its popularity, incredible productivity and a significant contribution to health outcomes. To accomplish this needs the contribution of all three levels of public health practitioner. This book provides us all with the necessary information, the ideas and the vision. I congratulate the authors.

David Colin-Thomé, MB.BS, FRCGP, FRCP, FFPH and FFGDP (Hon)
GP, Castlefields, Runcorn
National Clinical Director, DH England
Visiting Professor, Centre for Public Policy and Management,
Manchester University
Visiting Professor, School of Health, University of Durham

Foreword

2011 is just round the corner, the centenary of the introduction of health insurance which started the process not only of primary care but also of population-based care. The UK remains the only developed country in which primary care and population-based care are so closely entwined. In many other countries, insurance has taken a more direct role. Although insurance companies fund and manage high quality primary care, they do not have the same commitment to the population because there are often more than one insurance company providing for the population. In other countries, the cost of primary care is borne by patients themselves, often putting them into debt or depriving poorer communities of access to basic primary care. The universal nature of primary care provision in the NHS is one of its strongest features, as is the commitment to equitable population health.

Primary care in the UK is therefore a public health service as well as a clinical service in a way that is unique among developed countries.

One of the most useful pieces of advice that I was given by my first boss, John Warin, the Medical Officer of Health for Oxford was always to work towards my own redundancy, and this has been very useful advice. John Warin, like many other Medical Officers of Health, developed community health services, building on a long tradition going back, in the case of the School Health Service to 1908. All the time he was looking to develop primary care: investing in health visiting and then linking in health visitors to general practitioners; investing in district nurses and linking them to work with general practitioners; and, most significant of all, investing in health centres. These links are not always straightfoward but the general trend was unstoppable, and public health and primary care still work together to consider the needs of individuals and populations.

This book is very welcome because it describes the tools that can be used by people working in both public health and primary care in the UK. It is also relevant to other countries. Although our system is unusual at present, there is a trend in many other countries to link primary care and population-based care because it is no longer possible to allow every patient to move from one general practitioner to another, picking and choosing services. No country has the resources to afford this, and it does not provide high value health care.

This book, therefore, will be of great interest to people struggling to cope with the challenge of twenty-first century health care, the yawning gap, the Grand Canyon, between need and demand on one side and the resources that are available on the other.

J. A. Muir Gray, Kt, CBE, DSc, MD, FRCPSGlas, FCLIP
Programmes Director, National Screening Committee

Preface

This book is written for people working in primary care, who want to understand more about how they contribute to improving the health and health care of the populations that they serve, and for people working in public health, who want to understand the essential contribution of primary care to improving health. It sets out the nature, purpose and relevance of public health approaches to primary care practitioners and primary care organizations.

Primary care teams have had a long-established role in public health, providing preventive services to populations, through the registered list in general practice. This model has withstood multiple reconfigurations and reorganizations within the NHS and is the envy of many countries trying to create a public health system with primary care at its heart. There are clear differences in approach, with the inevitable conflicts between the rights of the individual set against the responsibility to ensure services are delivered fairly and equitably to whole populations. We explore this dilemma, showing how people working in primary care can cross the divide, to become part of the public health system, and in so doing are well placed to make a difference to the health of their populations.

We have sought to make this book relevant to people working in all parts of the UK and even internationally. This is not easy because with devolution within the UK, the systems for both public health and primary care are diverging, and public health is a political process which is closely tied into the policy context of the host country. We have therefore used policy in England to describe and illustrate public health processes in primary care, with the expectation that readers from other jurisdictions will be able to see the relevance to their situations.

The book is shaped around the public health process, and how it is applied within primary care. Chapters 1 and 2 review current policy and practice in public health and primary care respectively, reflecting on recent developments and future directions for both services. We describe in Chapter 3 the public health helix with people and their communities at the core of the public health process—and the helical motif is threaded through the book emphasizing the fact that the process is continuously evolving. Each time round the cycle the process has progressed and improved services for people and communities.

This attempts to simplify what is a tanglement of interconnected systems and should provide the reader with a clear conceptual framework to make sense of this complex world. The primary care system plays a central role in improving health of individuals and communities and we show how primary care practitioners contribute to this. Chapter 4 provides the essential tools for delivering public health within primary care. Inevitably, the chapter only briefly covers the vast array of tools and resources in daily use in public health practice. It concentrates on those tools of practical use for people working in primary care and it guides readers to where to obtain more information.

Chapters 5, 6 and 7 are the heart of the book. They take each of the three domains of public health practice—improving health, improving health care and protecting health—and reflect on the contribution that primary care organizations and primary care practitioners make to public health in each area. We illustrate the involvement and the inter-relationships with practical examples and with case studies to bring what could be a dry subject to life.

Chapter 8 looks at the education and the workforce in primary care and public health. There are several developments that are helping to bring the two disciplines closer. The medical and nursing Royal Colleges and the professional registering bodies now recognize public health as an essential thread in training. The emerging competency framework for NHS staff, and the job profiling arising from Agenda for Change (the new pay structure in the NHS) are allowing more flexibility and progression in careers, and blurring the boundaries between disciplines. Finally, in the epilogue (Chapter 9), we look to the future and reflect on those basic principles of public health and primary care that need to be protected and how the two disciplines need to evolve together to ensure that the public health potential of primary care is achieved in full.

A note on terminology

The terminology of primary care is somewhat confusing. Throughout this book, we have used the terms general practice and primary medical care to describe medical care provided by general practitioners (or family doctors elsewhere), and primary care for first contact care which is provided by a range of health care professionals including, nurses, dentists, pharmacists, optometrists, social workers and complementary therapists. Use of the term 'primary care' in a unitary way is increasingly inappropriate given the diversity of providers of first contact health services in the community.

For the most part, we refer to local bodies with commissioning and public health responsibilities as 'Primary Care Trusts'. The equivalents in other parts of the UK are local health boards (Wales), local health care cooperatives/NHS boards (Scotland) and health and social services trusts/health and social care groups (Northern Ireland). The term 'primary care organization' is used more generically to refer to all organizations, including general practices, that provide primary care.

Alison Hill
Siân Griffiths
Stephen Gillam

Acknowledgements

We are really grateful to Andy Chivers for reviewing the manuscript from the viewpoint of a primary care practitioner.

Contents

Authors

Stephen Gillam
General Practitioner, Luton;
Director, Public Health Teaching,
University of Cambridge Medical
School, UK; Visiting Professor,
University of Bedfordshire

Siân Griffiths
Professor and Director of School
of Public Health, The Chinese
University of Hong Kong,
Hong Kong

Alison Hill
Director, NHS Supporting Public
Health, Oxford, UK

Contributors

Jeremy Hawker
Head of Public Health Development,
Health Protection Agency,
London, UK

Tony Jewell
Chief Medical Officer, Welsh
Assembly Government, Cardiff, UK

Gillian Smith
Regional Epidemiologist, Health
Protection Agency, Birmingham, UK

Abbreviations and glossary

(See also an explanation of epidemiological terms on page 64–5 in Chapter 4)

CCDC: Consultant in Communicable Disease Control.

CHD: Coronary heart disease.

Chronic disease: an illness, such as heart disease or asthma, that is ongoing or recurring.

Chronic disease management: a system of care designed to improve patient care in long-term, ongoing illness.

Clinical audit: a quality improvement process that seeks to improve patient care and outcomes through systematic review of care against explicit criteria and the implementation of change.

Clinical governance: the framework that helps the NHS and other health care organizations provide safe and high quality care.

Community-oriented primary care: a strategy where elements of primary health care and public health are systematically developed and brought together in coordinated practice.

Director of Public Health (DPH): an executive member of a health authority or board, providing advocacy for public health across the community.

Environmental health: the theory and practice of assessing, correcting, controlling and preventing those factors in the environment that can potentially adversely affect the health of present and future generations.

Evaluation: a process that attempts to determine as systematically and objectively as possible the relevance, effectiveness and impact of activities in the light of their objectives (see Last JM, ed. A *Dictionary of Epidemiology*, 4th edn. Oxford: Oxford University Press, 2001).

Evidence-based health care/medicine/public health: systematic use of evidence derived from published research and other sources for management and practice.

Expressed needs: needs expressed by action, e.g. visiting a doctor.

Felt needs: what people consider and/or say they need

Foundation Trusts: health care organizations which are part of the NHS but have a significant amount of managerial and financial freedom.

General Medical Services (GMS): the contract which covers the pay arrangement between the Primary Care Trust (PCT) or the Health Board (in Scotland) and a General Practitioner (GP) practice.

GOBI-FFF: low cost primary care interverntions of growth monitoring, oral rehydration, breast feeding, immunization; female education, family spacing, food supplements.

GP: general practitioner (family doctor).

GP fundholding: a practice which manages a budget for its practice staff, certain hospital referrals, drug costs, community nursing services and management costs. It was introduced in 1991 and abolished in 1998.

Health: the extent to which an individual or a group is able to realize aspirations and satisfy needs, and to change or cope with the environment. Health is a resource for everyday life, not the objective of living; it is a positive concept, emphasizing social and personal resources as well as physical capabilities. Your health is related to how much you feel your potential, to be a meaningful part of the society in which you find yourself, is adequately realized (see Last JM, ed. A *Dictionary of Epidemiology*, 4th edn. Oxford: Oxford University Press, 2001).

Health Action Zones: partnerships between the NHS, local authorities, the voluntary and private sectors and local communities which aim to reduce health inequalities between rich and poor.

Healthcare Commission: a body in England that assures, monitors and helps improve the quality of patient care by undertaking reviews of clinical governance (www.healthcarecommission.org.uk accessed 14 October 2006).

Health Development Agency (HDA): a special health authority established in 2000 to develop the evidence base to improve health and reduce health inequalities. It was incorporated into NICE (see below) in April 2005.

Health equity: fair distribution of health or health care resources or opportunities according to population need or an equal share of resource for an equal need.

Health impact assessment (HIA): an assessment process to look at the impact on health of government policies or other actions, completed or projected.

Health improvement: the theory and practice of promoting the health of populations by influencing lifestyle and socio-economic, physical and cultural environment through methods of health promotion, directed towards populations, communities and individuals.

Health inequality: the gap in health status, and in access to health services, between different social classes and ethnic groups and between populations in different geographical areas.

Healthy Living Centres: a lottery-funded programme that provided initiatives, partnerships and networks in deprived areas, which focus on health in its broadest sense, providing opportunities to improve quality of life and enable people to achieve their full potential.

Health outcome: health status, sometimes related to the effects of health care or other interventions.

Health promotion: the process of enabling people to increase control over and improve their health. As well as covering actions aimed at strengthening people's skills and capabilities, it also includes actions directed towards changing social, environmental conditions to prevent or to improve their impact on individual and public health.

Health protection: the branch of public health that deals with the control of disease related to infectious and environmental hazards.

Health visitor: qualified and registered nurse or midwife who has undertaken further (post-registration) training in order to be able to work as a member of the primary health care team. The role of the health visitor is about the promotion of health and the prevention of illness in all age groups.

HPA: Health Protection Agency.

HIV/AIDS: human immunodeficiency virus, acquired immunodeficiency syndrome.

Life expectancy: an estimate of the average number of years a newborn baby would survive if he or she experienced the particular area's age-specific mortality rates for that time period throughout his or her life.

Local Area Agreements (LAAs): agreements between government, the local authority and its major delivery partners in an area (working through the Local Strategic Partnerships). They simplify the number of additional funding streams from central government going into an area, help join up public services more effectively and allow greater flexibility for local solutions to local circumstances.

Local Strategic Partnerships (LSPs): bodies based on local authority boundaries, bringing together public, private, community and voluntary sectors, tasked with tackling those issues which require the involvement of several agencies to solve. The LSPs support their local authorities' community strategies, and the new initiatives called Local Area Agreements (see above).

National Institute for Health and Clinical Excellence (NICE): NICE is the UK independent organization responsible for providing national guidance on the promotion of good health and the prevention and treatment of ill health (http://www.nice.org.uk/ accessed 14 October 2006).

National Service Framework (NSF) (UK): NSFs set national standards and define service models for a specific service or care group, put in place programmes to support implementation, and establish performance measures against which progress within an agreed time scale will be measured.

NGO: non-governmental organization.

NHS: National Health Service.

NHS Direct: a special health authority responsible for delivering all NHS Direct services in England including NHS Direct telephone service, NHS Direct Online website, NHS Direct Interactive digital TV, and NHS Direct self-help guide.

Normative needs: needs as defined by a health professional.

Payment by results: a system for paying trusts linked to activity and adjusted for case mix using a pre-agreed national tariff.

PCO: primary care organization

Personal Medical Services (PMS): schemes intended to give GPs, nurses and community trusts the opportunity to provide new, more flexible ways of offering primary care services that are sensitive to local needs, in particular meeting the needs of deprived communities and improving patient access to services.

Practice-based commissioning: practices are provided with the resources and support to become more involved in commissioning decisions. They receive information on how their patients use health services which they can use for the redesign of services.

Prevention: primary, secondary and tertiary (see below).

Primary care: see primary health care.

Primary Care Trust (PCT): local NHS health authorities in England charged with improving health, and commissioning health care.

Primary health care: first contact care provided by a range of health care professionals, nurses, dentists, pharmacists, optometrists and complementary therapists.

Primary medical care: medical care provided by GPs.

Primary prevention: aims to promote wellbeing and to prevent the onset of disease by reducing risk factors in the population either through changes in behaviour and lifestyle, or through changes in the environment supported by appropriate public policies and health education.

Public health: the science and art of preventing disease, prolonging life and promoting health through the organized efforts of society. Public health practice is the emphasis in this book, while public health may also be considered as a discipline or a social institution.

Public health practitioner: in this book, includes anyone working in the broad field of public health, neither defined by formal qualifications nor restricted to a professional group.

Quality and Outcomes Framework (QOF): a system for payment of GPs in the NHS. It was introduced as part of the new General Medical Services NHS contract in April 2004.

RCT: randomized controlled trial.

Risk: the probability that a particular adverse event occurs during a stated period of time, or results from a particular challenge. It can never be reduced to zero.

SARS: severe acute respiratory syndrome.

Screening: the systematic application of a test or inquiry to identify individuals at sufficient risk of a specific disorder to benefit from further investigation or direct preventive action among persons who have not sought medical attention on account of symptoms of that disorder.

Secondary prevention: aims to halt the progress of an established disease through early diagnosis and treatment. Screening asymptomatic people for a disease is one example of secondary prevention backed up by counselling, health education and effective treatment.

Stakeholders: persons or organizations with an interest that may affect the outcome of an activity. Responses to stakeholders may include collaboration, involvement, monitoring or defence.

STI: sexually transmitted infection.

Surveillance: the ongoing, systematic collection, collation and analysis of data, and the prompt dissemination of the resulting information to those who need to know so that an action can result.

Tertiary prevention: aims to prevent disease progression and attendant suffering after a disease is clinically obvious and a diagnosis established.

TB: tuberculosis.

Walk-in Centres: these provide access to local NHS services, information and treatment without needing an appointment. They do not replace local GP or hospital services but complement them.

WHO: World Health Organization.

1

What is public health?

This chapter describes the historical basis of public health, its impact on current structures and relationships between public health and primary care.

We review recent policies in England which have contributed to shaping modern public health practice, recognizing that devolution has led to the development of individual public health policies in the four countries within the UK.

We go on to describe some of the concepts used in shaping policy which are relevant to understanding the public health approach:

- The three domains of practice
- Life course approach
- Individual and population approaches
- Primary, secondary and tertiary prevention
- Pathways of care and National Service Frameworks.

Public health is concerned with the health of populations and takes account of all the factors which influence the health of both individuals and groups of people. For primary care practitioners, it can seem confusingly broad and diffuse. This brief review of its historical origins aims for a better understanding of public health and its links with primary care.

The historical context of public health

Ancient roots

An awareness of the need for clean water, clean air, a decent place to live and a holistic approach to health is not new. In ancient Greece, the Hippocratic essays on 'Air, Waters and Places' recognized the influence of environment, climate, soil, nutrition, water and way of life[1] on health. In 384 BC, Aristotle was writing about the well-being of the whole person in his Eudamonia.

In the middle ages, municipal authorities struggled to provide clean drinking water and keep the streets clean, as evidenced by visits to many archaeological and historic sites. Medieval communities had systems for disease prevention, sanitary supervision and general protection of the health of local communities. Examples include the paving of Parisian streets in 1185 and the regulations stipulating that Florentine markets should be swept clean every evening to remove bones and other rubbish.

By the eighteenth century, there was growing recognition that the state had responsibilities for the health of the people. In Germany, Johann Peter Frank, a medical pioneer of public health, suggested the creation of health police, while early in the nineteenth century Jeremy Bentham proposed his constitutional code to deal with environmental sanitation, communicable disease and medical administration. Among other significant figures in the development of British public health, John Simon stated in 1858 that 'sanitary neglect is mistaken parsimony ... The physical strength of a nation is among the chief factors of national prosperity'[1]. Sir Edwin Chadwick, motivated by similar economic arguments, was the prime mover in getting legislation passed. His report on the Sanitary Conditions of the Labouring Population led to the 1848 Public Health Act and the establishment of Medical Officers of Health (MOsH) with population-based responsibility for health.

The first MOH

The first MOH, William Henry Duncan, was appointed in 1848 to work in Liverpool. He found himself dealing with appalling urban housing conditions, the product of the rapid growth of the populations in the newly industrialized cities. One-third of the working class population in his patch were living in narrow, airless courts. Descriptions of people coming from the countryside sleeping 30 in a room, many of them in underground cellars, were not uncommon, so it was hardly surprising that the death rate in Liverpool was the highest in the country. According to William Farr, 'so unfavourable to infant life are the unsanitary conditions of the large towns especially Liverpool that not only is the mortality at some months of age twice as high as it is in the healthier districts but at seven months and upwards it is three times'[2]. Duncan used his sanitary powers as MOH to improve housing and living conditions, a major contribution to raising life expectancy and quality of life among the poor. He relied heavily on the use of biostatistics to describe his population. Statistics were also one of the key tools used by Farr's close colleague, Florence Nightingale. Often better known for her key role in developing nursing than her statistical flair, her contribution to understanding and promoting population health led to her recognition by the influential Statistical Society.

The Broad Street Pump

The best known story of Victorian public health concerns John Snow. Even now there is a pub in London's Soho marking the site in Broad Street of the famous pump. Snow applied his theory that the spread of cholera was borne through water rather than 'miasma'. He used basic epidemiological research to persuade the local authorities to remove the pump handle which stemmed the epidemic.

Box 1.1 The Broad Street Pump

Asiatic cholera first hit England in late 1831, and nothing seemed to be effective in containing it. An outbreak in London in 1854 provided John Snow with the chance to test his theory, based on careful observation and mapping of previous outbreaks, that cholera 'always commences with disturbances of the functions of the alimentary canal' and is spread by a poison passed from victim to victim through sewage-tainted water. Through a unique piece of detective work, he systematically traced the consumers of water from the pump in Broad Street, Soho as the source of the local epidemic by mapping deaths to the source of water and showing that there was a single source of polluted water. He had noted that with the naked eye one could see that water from the pump contained 'white, flocculent particles'. He took his findings to the Board of Guardians of St James's Parish who, although they were reluctant to believe him, agreed to the removal of the pump handle. This dramatically stopped the spread of cholera.

Early public health practice was much concerned with the environmental factors which contribute to ill health, particularly of the poor. While doctors, civil servants and legislators all played a role, architects and engineers also made key contributions. For example, Joseph Bazalgette built the London sewer system following the 'Big Stink' of 1858 when the Houses of Parliament became so smelly that the members demanded action. In response to politicians' concerns, his sewer network diverted raw sewage downstream, a masterpiece of engineering which is still admired.

Understanding infectious disease

Public health relies on standardized measures to describe health status, particularly death rates (see Chapter 4). In the latter half of the nineteenth century, death rates in England from infectious disease for those aged between 24 and 40 years dropped by 60 per cent. At the same time, the infant mortality rate dropped by 18 per cent. Such changes indicated that health was improving as the environment in which people lived improved.

The turn of the nineteenth century was accompanied by a rapid growth in scientific understanding of the microbial causes of communicable diseases and their treatment. The work of Pasteur, Cohn, Koch and others laid the foundation of current microbiology, with a rapid series of discoveries linking bacteria with diseases and early understanding of immunity.

Developing personal public health services

With improving social conditions—better housing, better working conditions, a concern for education—the focus of public health shifted to the development of personal preventive services. Maternal and child welfare became a priority. As early as 1854 in France there was interest in promoting mother/child health through special programmes which included antenatal care and the supply of clean milk to babies. In England, legislation such as the 1902 Midwives Act, the 1906 provision of school meals legislation and the 1918 Maternity and Child Welfare Acts provided the impetus for investment in midwifery, health visiting and school nursing as part of the community-based public health service. Mass vaccination and immunization were introduced, and the emphasis on disease prevention increased. Public health services such as these form a core part of today's public health services in lower and middle income countries.

The minority report of the 1909 Poor Law Commission, largely written by Beatrice Webb, proposed creating a state medical service which unified public health authorities with the poor law medical services to be administered as part of the social security system. The 1929 Local Government Act increased hospital resources of county and borough councils. Finally, in 1948, the National Health Service (NHS) established a comprehensive health system for improving the people's health through the prevention, diagnosis and treatment of illness.

The public health services and MOsH continued to be outside the NHS in local government until 1974. Up to this time, every year local authority councillors were given a report on the state of their population's health through the MOH's annual report. This report would describe annual progress in the areas for which the MOH was responsible and account to them as locally elected representatives. These responsibilities included surveillance and control of communicable disease, environmental health, and social and community services. For example, the 1973 report for the City of Oxford[3] describes how the public health department had assumed responsibility not only for infectious disease control, housing and food safety, but also for community nursing services, dental health, immunization and the development of health centres where health visitors, midwives, practice nurses and social workers were working alongside local family doctors. In summary, by 1968, MOsH had a "smoothly running empire", managing community nursing services, social work services, the aftercare of people who were mentally ill or handicapped, the ambulances and the child and school health services[4].

Public health joins the NHS

The NHS re-organization of 1974 brought together under one organization the three strands of modern public health—health protection, medical management of health services, and health improvement and promotion. This was the first of a series of structural changes which saw the separation, albeit temporary, of public health from primary care as the focus of public health shifted to management of NHS resources at the expense of both engagement in primary care and concern with determinants of health. During this time, the NHS introduced the philosophy of the market with the initiation of the purchaser–provider split and growing managerialism. With their population-based skills and understanding of organizations, many public health specialists focused more on the acute sector and on the contracting process than on promoting health, particularly through working with primary care. However, in recent years, there has been a shift back to the wider role and local responsibilities of the Director of Public Health (DsPH) and their team. There has also been a growing understanding by health care professionals and others in primary care of the impact of social and economic conditions on the health of patients and their families and the role they as health care professionals can play.

Public health challenges

The 1974 move into the NHS confused the roles of public health practitioners. Relationships with local government were weakened and the focus became the management of health services within inadequate budgets. The managerial reforms of the 1980s and the separation of 'purchasers' of health services from their 'providers' left many public health professionals perceived by primary care practitioners as mere administrators, often responsible for refusing funding for a new medical service. Donald Acheson's report on 'Public Health in England'[5], however, helped to revitalize the public health role particularly in relation to communicable disease control. He promulgated a definition of public health (derived from Winslow) which is still commonly used: 'The science and art of preventing disease, prolonging life and promoting health through the organised efforts of society'.

This definition of public health chimed with the Ottawa Charter[6], later adopted as a cornerstone for practice by the public health community. The Charter identified five key areas for action:

- Building healthy public policy
- Creating supportive environments
- Strengthening community action
- Developing personal skills
- Re-orienting health services towards prevention and a holistic approach.

Coupled with the Alma Ata declaration[7], the Charter echoed the historic roots of public health, that is the important and interactive roles of government, communities and individuals alongside the health care sector in promoting good health and preventing disease.

This approach also underscores the essentially different perspectives of public health and clinical practice. Whilst the clinician is faced on a daily basis with patients with disease-related problems, public health practitioners are faced with the challenges of systems for health and health care. Box 1.2 is a well known illustration, if somewhat overstated, of these different approaches.

Box 1.2 Public health: the upstream approach

Health workers can be likened to a lifesaver on the bank of a river: every so often a drowning person is swept along past them. The lifesaver dives in to the rescue, retrieves the 'patient' and resuscitates them. Just as they have finished another casualty appears alongside. So busy and involved are the lifesavers in all of this rescue work that they have no time to walk upstream and see why it is that so many people are falling in the river. The public health worker moves upstream to see what is the cause of falling into the river and takes action to prevent people falling into the river in the first place

Ashton and Seymour[8], p. vii

The breadth of public health was once more highlighted in the Bangkok Charter[9] which states that the promotion of health is:

- central to the global development agenda
- a core responsibility for all of government
- a key focus of communities and civil society
- a requirement for good corporate practice.

The Charter shifts from the stereotypical portrayal of multinational companies such as MacDonald's and Coca Cola as solely a health threat to recognizing the need to work in partnership with the corporate sector to create healthier environments in which individuals can make choices. The values underpinning the Charter are those of social justice, gender and health equity, respect for diversity and human dignity, and the search for peace and security.

While many countries have now signed up to this declaration, the importance of public health systems has not always been fully recognized. By the 1970s, universal concerns about clean water, a healthy environment and improving living conditions of society were not seen as priorities for investment. In a view dominated by complacency within developed countries, it was mistakenly assumed that basic issues such as the control of communicable disease and healthy living conditions were resolved or at least resolvable. Health care was all important, and the majority of available resources were being committed to hospital-based care. Prevention was receiving little attention from either politicians or the press, and many public health systems remained underdeveloped. Indeed, in 1963, the US Surgeon General wrote: 'it might be possible with interventions such as antimicrobials and vaccines to close the book on infectious diseases and shift public health resources to chronic diseases'[10].

However, events in recent years have increased recognition of the importance of public health services and approaches. The events of 9/11 reawakened an awareness of the importance of public health not only for those who specialize in population health science but more importantly to a wide range of sectors in society[11]. Natural disasters and terrorist bombings have highlighted the global responsibility of coordinated early responses and of rebuilding communities in the longer term. The experience of SARS (severe acute respiratory syndrome) and the threat of newly emerging infections such as avian 'flu are a constant reminder of the importance of the need for robust systems for disease surveillance and preparedness to combat communicable diseases. The threat of an epidemic directly threatens the economic well-being of all countries. Meanwhile, in some parts of the world, most notably sub-Saharan Africam HIV/AIDS (human immunodeficiency virus/acquired immunodeficiency syndrome), the control of malaria, and the problems of resistant tuberculosis (TB) are not only the major health issues but are also the economic ones.

However, economic and social challenges are not only posed by the threat of epidemics of communicable disease but also by those of increasingly affluent lifestyles. Tobacco, obesity and stress contribute to a massive economic and social burden, storing up problems for future generations. Many countries in transition, particularly those with rapidly developing economies such as China and India, face the 'double whammy' of poverty-related diseases as well as those associated with growing affluence. The World Health Organization[12] have estimated that 40 per cent of the global burden of disease is due to preventable causal factors (see Box 1.3). The list demonstrates the challenges not only of poverty but also of affluence.

Box 1.3 The global burden of disease

Forty per cent of global deaths are due to:

- ◆ Child and maternal underweight
- ◆ Unsafe sex
- ◆ High blood pressure
- ◆ Tobacco
- ◆ Alcohol
- ◆ Unsafe water
- ◆ Poor sanitation and hygiene
- ◆ High cholesterol
- ◆ Indoor smoke from solid fuels
- ◆ Iron deficiency
- ◆ Overweight/obesity

These are the factors which contribute to chronic non-communicable diseases which are now the major cause of death and disability worldwide. It is estimated that over 35 million people died from chronic non-communicable diseases in 2005, double the number from all infectious diseases (including HIV/AIDS, TB and malaria), maternal and perinatal conditions, and nutritional deficiencies combined. Chronic diseases cause death not only in old age but prematurely amongst the middle aged[13].

Addressing the non-communicable disease challenge needs us to take account of the various factors which predispose to ill health (see Fig. 1.1).

Without concerted action at all levels, the UK will not be exempt from the threats facing the rest of the world. 'Choosing Health' estimated that in a 50 year period, affluent lifestyles reflected in increasing obesity rates will increase the incidence of coronary heart disease-related morbidity and that by 2023 there will have been a 54 per cent increase in type 2 diabetes[14] (see Fig. 1.2).

The need for public health systems

To address the challenges of both chronic long-term disease and communicable disease, we need good public health systems and we need to understand the

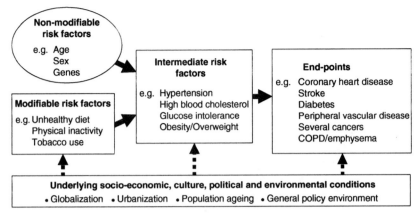

80 per cent of heart disease, stroke, type 2 diabetes
40 per cent of cancer would be prevented

Fig. 1.1 Non-communicable diseases are preventable.

relationships between public health, with its focus starting on populations, and primary health care with its focus starting with individuals, which we explore further later in the book.

This relationship does not need to be polarized between two perspectives but to meld them into an appropriate response to the needs of any individual or patient for whom the social situation is as relevant as clinical symptoms.

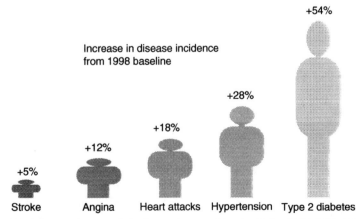

Fig. 1.2 Estimated impact of the increasing trend in obesity by 2023 (UK). Adapted from 'Choosing Health'[14]. Projections should be interpreted with caution, as they assume current trends will continue unabated.

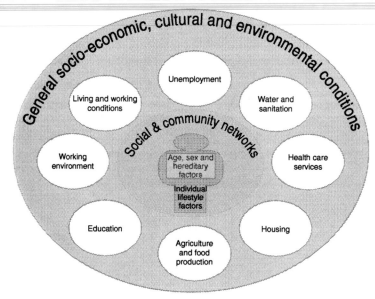

Fig. 1.3 Factors affecting health.

This needs us to take account of the broad range of concerns, illustrated in Fig. 1.3, which are relevant to healthy lives for individuals.

Underpinning this approach is the need for partnership at many levels: government at all levels, the corporate sector, communities and academics, as well as the health care sector including primary care. Primary health care has a key role to play in creating synergy to deliver better outcomes from the health-care delivery system[15]. We describe partnership working in more detail in Chapter 3.

Public health policy and its interface with primary care

Public health policy

Context

In the earlier part of this chapter, we have described the history and broader context of public health and its relationship to primary health care as well as the need to position primary care within a broader conceptual framework than providing care to individual patients. To develop the context further and to understand better modern public health practice, we have reviewed the background both to policy development and to the structures for delivery. Here we have focused on England, recognizing that there are different policies and structures in the four countries within the UK, not to mention international examples. However, the underlying principles and issues to be addressed are, in the main, common, and English public health policy is recognized as being well developed.

Background

From our brief historical description, the interplay between developments in primary care, and population measures to promote and protect health are evident. Whilst health visitors were originally public health workers in local government organizations, they are now key members of primary care teams. Social care, once in the domain of the MOH, is now a main concern of primary care organizations (PCOs), in which DsPH now work. Government policy and the structural changes which influenced the early twentieth century provision of school health, health visiting and midwifery services continue in the twenty-first century to influence the dynamics of the public health roles of the primary care teams. Whilst the focus of the Thatcher governments was on managerialism, drawing public health specialists away from their local government roots and tying them more closely into the day-to-day running of health care where they were clearly identified with the role of purchasing health authorities, the subsequent Labour administration refocused on the wider determinants of health. They re-established the links between public health and local government and drew public health closer to primary care. Emphasis has been placed on the health improvement role of PCOs, incentivizing prevention through the GP contract and bringing DsPH back into community-based organizations. The policy framework which initiated such moves includes structural White Papers, one of which is worth specific comment.

Organizational White Papers

'**Shifting the Balance of Power**'[16], published in 2002, brought PCOs and public health closer together. Primary Care Trusts (PCTs) became responsible for three main tasks:

- Improving the health of the community
- Securing the provision of services
- Integrating health and social care.

The plan was for each PCT to have a DsPH supported by a strong public health team to focus on improving health, preventing serious illness and reducing inequalities in the populations they served. Recognizing that this would severely stretch the capacity of the public health specialist workforce, the DsPH and their teams were to be part of a *public health network* of skills, knowledge and experience in every local area, with networks designed according to local needs[17] (see Chapter 4 for a discussion on understanding needs).

To deliver the public health agenda, PCOs needed a range of skills and appropriately trained staff which included not only public health specialists, needed for their analytical and organizational skills, but public health practitioners such as health visitors and school nurses to deliver health promotion and disease prevention programmes, as well as GPs with a special interest, social workers, pharmacists and dentists who all had a role to play in prevention.

The huge agenda in commissioning acute care faced by many PCTs, compounded by the lack of trained public health specialists, meant progress was patchy and fragmented. Progress was made in some areas, for example enhanced working with local government through joint appointments of DsPH between PCTs and their local authorities. This model is one which gained favour in Wales and has been easier to achieve in parts of the country where boundaries between PCTs and their local authorities were co-terminous. In successful models, some local councils and PCTs have even pooled resources to create joint units, with shared membership of public health teams. These teams enable closer joint working between PCTs and local government, and play a key role in bridging the different agendas relevant to better health for their shared population[18]. One good example of joint working at a local level between PCTs and local authority partners is the development of Local Strategic Partnerships (LSPs) and Local Area Agreements (LAAs) (see Chapter 3). LSPs are plans which local government is required to produce about how they will act on their responsibility for the social, environmental and economic factors which impact on health in their patch. Figure 1.4 shows diagrammatically how

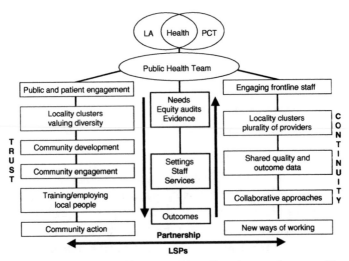

Fig. 1.4 The roles of public health teams with staff, patients and communities (from Drinkwater[19]).

the public health team can bridge the different cultures of local government and the NHS to achieve effective partnership.

Public health policies relevant to primary care practice

In addition to structural reforms, there have been four milestones of public health policy in England:

- Saving Lives: Our Healthier Nation
- The Acheson Review
- The Wanless reports
- Choosing Health: Making Healthy Choices Easier.

'Saving Lives: Our Healthier Nation'[20]   This is the first public health White Paper of the Labour government and was published in 1998, setting the new direction of public health policy. Its key points are summarized in Box 1.4.

Box 1.4 Key elements of 'Saving Lives'

- Focused on reducing inequalities in health
- Addressed the wider determinants of health
- Introduced health impact assessment
- Established Public Health Observatories to monitor health
- Set targets for cancer, coronary heart disease, stroke, accidents, mental health
- Emphasized partnerships especially through primary care, health improvement programmes, healthy living centres, health action zones
- Widened the public health workforce to include multidisciplinary specialist role

---

Inequalities: the Acheson review   Addressing social inequalities and their impact on health has become a main policy initiative not only in the UK and Europe, but in many other societies. The value placed on equity as well as the inter-relationship between health and economic prosperity are reflected in the work of world-renowned figures such as Amartya Sen, Jeffrey Sachs and Sir Michael Marmot.

Sir Donald Acheson, building on the tenets of the Black report[21], reviewed evidence of what was needed to reduce health inequalities in the UK[22]. The report highlighted the relatively small contribution of health services to health status and the key contributions of education, housing, employment and income.

Health inequalities are important not only because people are living longer in the UK but because increasing length of life is unevenly distributed between social groups (Fig. 1.5). The extra years are not necessarily healthy years. A boy born in Manchester in 2005 has a life expectancy 8 years shorter than a boy born in Dorset. The health differential between the north and south of England is a consistent finding in studies of coronary heart disease and associated health behaviours.

Active steps to tackle inequalities have been a main plank of health and social policy[23,24]. The UK government made reducing inequalities a key theme for its European Presidency[25], and many countries are concerned with the need to address not only equity (fair distribution and access to services) but also inequalities or disparities (differences in the health status of groups of the population).

Two national targets were set in 2001 focusing on increasing healthy life expectancy and reducing infant mortality. Targets at national and local (PCT) level have been further refined to include targets to reduce tobacco smoking and teenage pregnancy, as well as to reduce obesity. Whilst it is easy to set targets, it is more difficult to achieve change. Indicators which reflect interventions which could most reduce inequalities include teenage pregnancy, road accident casualties, educational achievement, homelessness, and fruit and vegetable consumption. Recent work has shown that progress is being made in all these areas, although the gap between 'haves' and 'have nots' remains to be closed.

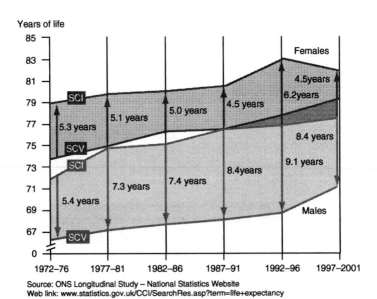

Source: ONS Longitudinal Study – National Statistics Website
Web link: www.statistics.gov.uk/CCI/SearchRes.asp?term=life+expectancy

Fig. 1.5 Life expectancy at birth by social class and sex. Department of Health (2006) *Health Profile of England*. London: Department of Health. Crown copyright.

At PCT level, DsPH, through their annual reports, equity audits (see Chapter 4 and 6) and working with local government, promote these priorities and monitor progress. At practice level, the new General Medical Services (GMS) contract provides incentives to GPs and practices actively to engage in promoting healthier lifestyles and reducing inequalities (See Chapter 2).

Role of the Chancellor: the Wanless reports   The work on reducing health inequalities underscores the potential impact of government policies from other departments, particularly the Treasury. It is the Chancellor of the Exchequer who has led the drive to eradicate child poverty through policies such as Family Tax Credit, the minimum wage, and Surestart (http://www.surestart.gov.uk/). Such commitment was exemplified by commissioning Sir Derek Wanless'[26] whose report sought to answer the question: 'What resources will be needed in 20 years time to provide high quality health services in the UK?' Three scenarios were proposed:

'*Slow uptake*' where little changed from the UK's historic path.

'*Solid progress*' which meant succeeding with announced plans while enhancing the productivity of the health care sector, measured in terms of throughput and efficiency

'*Fully engaged*' which would see further life expectancy improvements (to 81.6 years for men and 85.5 years for women) and significant further engagement in prevention.

His first report encouraged government to think more about the health care system and standards, and it is widely credited as the catalyst for the extra investment in the NHS made in 2002. Wanless' second report[27] reviewed the state of public health and how to implement the 'fully engaged' scenario. This scenario placed more emphasis on prevention and on greater public health capacity and capability—more people to do things better. It also stressed the need for a greater focus on the use of evidence and involving patients and the public in decision making about their health. To do this, better use of new technology and information systems are needed, underpinned by relevant research programmes and supported by better measurement tools[28].

The third chapter of the report discusses in detail the role of PCOs stating in its conclusion that 'PCTs as the main NHS organization responsible for improving health need appropriate incentives and performance management to enable them to prioritise public health issues and to work in partnership with local players to achieve this'. The roles of primary care team members and the opportunities of the new GMS contract and Quality and Outcomes Framework are also discussed.

This second Wanless report is also credited with stimulating a further public health White Paper, 'Choosing Health: Making Healthy Choices Easier'[14].

'Choosing Health' 'Choosing Health' focused on promoting healthy choices for individuals and providing support for lifestyle change, emphasisng the key role of primary care.

'Choosing Health' emphasized 'individual choice within a supportive environment'. Sensitive to media criticism, this White Paper was keen to emphasize that the role of government was not to create a nanny state but to promote the role of the individual and their choice for a healthy life. It focused on initiatives to support personal health, making children a priority. Initiatives included expanding the roles of school nurses, linked to PCTs, whose role was to coordinate a 'whole school' approach to health which focuses on diet, particularly school meals, and physical activity. Local authorities (district councils) were given the lead in creating local partnerships and for working with local voluntary groups and businesses. Emphasis was placed on providing extra support to deprived communities to tackle health inequalities.

PCOs were identified as key players in this agenda, not only as a community partner but through the work of staff at many levels. However, sustaining momentum for these initiatives in the face of organizational change and budget deficits poses a challenge for PCOs.

Box 1.5 Key objectives of Choosing Health[14]

- To reduce the numbers of people who smoke—building on current progress
- To reduce obesity—with new action with a focus on children
- To increase physical activity by increasing more opportunities
- To promote support for sensible drinking of alcohol
- To improve sexual health with investment in new campaigns and services particularly addressing sexually transmitted infections and implementing the sexual health strategy
- To improve mental health and well-being, crucial to good physical health
- To develop the public health workforce

Public health practice: underlying concepts and the interface with primary care

Whilst history determines the context we work in and policy reflects the direction of the government, the synergy of public health and primary care relies on local cooperation. Structural change and new policies exert a top-down influence but are often unheeded in everyday practice. Some examples of how public health can contribute to primary care in practice are given in Box 1.6.

Box 1.6 Examples of how public health can contribute to primary care

Health surveillance, monitoring and analysis

DsPH annual reports can be used to make better use of computerized data; utilizing information and intelligence from across the primary care team to describe the practice population, to identify unmet need and assist planning.

Investigation of disease outbreaks, epidemics and risks to health

Immunization is a responsibility of primary care, but public health specialists can provide support in outbreaks of communicable disease such as meningitis or TB. The threats of avian ' flu, debates about prophylaxis with Tamiflu and the emergency arrangements should a pandemic occur are all issues in which public health specialists in health protection can provide support to local practices and PCOs.

Health promotion and disease prevention programmes

The experience of the smoking cessation service provides a good example of the synergy between public health expertise and primary care team delivery. While clinicians provide or refer for advice, public health specialists review improvements, monitor targets and devise effective ways of delivering services particularly to hard to reach groups.

Working with local communities to improve health and reduce inequalities

PCTs have close relationships with local authorities who take the lead on addressing the broader determinants of health. The NHS planning framework National Standards: Local Action expects them to deliver reduced obesity, lower sexual infection rates, reduced smoking rates and a reduction in health inequalities. Public health expertise can help provide information on effective interventions, to evaluate local initiatives and support overall design of initiatives delivered to patients by PCT members.

Ensuring effective performance of health services

Public health approaches to effective health service planning, including effective use of evidence, can support practice-based commissioning. In addition, the new contracts for GPs, pharmacists and dentists can all be used to incentivize the engagement of primary care professionals in prevention.

Engaging in research at local level or participating in wider research networks

Utilizing both epidemiological and other skills to understand better the health of the population can support better understanding of local health needs.

Underpinning concepts

As described above, there are many opportunities for synergy at a local level between public health (population) and primary care (individual) approaches to be shared within PCOs. Effective collaborative approaches and deeper understanding will be underpinned by considering and sharing some key concepts:

1. The domains of public health practice
2. Lifecourse approach
3. Population and individual approaches
4. The hierarchy of prevention
5. Pathway of care.

Concept 1: the three domains of public health practice

As we have described earlier in this chapter, the historical origins of public health lie in the challenges of promoting and protecting the public's health. Three historically rooted pathways—health protection, health improvement and improving health systems—are drawn together within the three domains of public health practice[29] (http://www.fphm.org.uk/) (Fig. 1.6). Public health delivery relies on public health programmes which bring together all key contributors. We will describe this approach in Chapter 3.

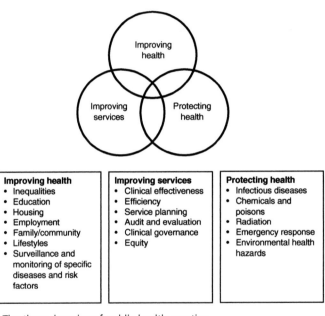

Fig. 1.6 The three domains of public health practice.

By identifying these three domains of public health as areas of practice, underpinned by good information, epidemiology and biostatistics as well as an understanding of law and ethical issues and good academic research, it is possible to describe not only who might be involved in a public health programme but how individuals can contribute from their different roles and perspectives. This includes both members of public health teams and members of primary care teams in delivering, for example, public health programmes to reduce tobacco related harm, prevent teen pregnancy/support teen mothers, reduce obesity and promote healthy ageing. Table 1.1 illustrates the application of the three domains to the health of older people.

The concept of the three domains of practice underpins our approach and is further developed in Chapters 5, 6 and 7.

Table 1.1 Applying the three domains of public health to ageing

Health improvement	Physical activity—falls prevention
	Healthy and adequate diet
	Social support
	Housing
	Safe neighbourhoods
	Transport
	Lifelong learning
	Pensions/benefits advice
Health protection	Flu vaccine
	Hospital control of infection to reduce MRSA infection
Quality of health/ social/care services	Community support
	Evidence-based care for common conditions such as stroke
	Patient-centred approach for maintaining long term conditions, e.g. diabetes
	Ensuring strategies support non-discriminatory access to care
	Providing evidence-based information for patients
	Working between local authorities and primary care to promote greater integration of services

Concept 2: lifecourse approach

The risk of developing chronic disease accumulates with age and is influenced by factors acting at all stages of the life span. The impact of social and biological influences throughout life is both cumulative and interactive, and early life factors are particularly important in creating a predisposition to chronic disease in later years. Functional capacity such as cardiovascular output, lung function and muscular strength increase in childhood and peak in early adulthood, eventually followed by a decline with a rate that is largely determined by factors related to adult lifestyle such as smoking, physical inactivity, unhealthy nutrition and excessive alcohol consumption, as well as external and environmental factors. However, the degree of decline can be moderated through healthy lifestyles and effective health care and may be reversible at any age through individual actions and public policy measures. It is therefore important to secure growth and development in early life, and to maintain the highest possible level of function in adult life, as well as maintaining quality of life in older age through independent living and preventing disability in later years. This approach is described as the lifecourse approach and underpins many of the epidemiological studies which inform policy[30].

Concept 3: individual or population approaches?

One of the tensions in primary care and public health practice arises from the different outcomes sought by the different parties. Whilst for some the long-term investment in promoting health takes priority, for others the shorter term rewards of curing illness are foremost in their minds. The results of promoting health may not be immediately apparent for several generations, whereas treatment brings observable benefits. Clinicians treat individuals, public health strategies seek to improve the health of the entire population. Gains that are substantial at a population level may have only limited benefit for an individual and vice versa. For example, improving nutrition through promoting healthier foods or reducing exposure to tobacco smoke by banning smoking in public places may help a population, but treatment to reduce hypertension will directly help an individual.

Using the example of raised blood cholesterol as a public health problem, we know that between 15 and 20 per cent of people in the UK have raised blood cholesterol levels and are thus at increased risk of cardiovascular disease. For these individuals, their level of risk depends on how much the cholesterol is raised, their genetic propensity to heart disease and what other risk factors they have. Should treatment be targeted at the small proportion (5 per cent) of people at highest risk? Or should everybody in the population be encouraged to make changes in their lifestyle so that the average level of blood cholesterol is lowered and every person's risk is lowered by a small amount? The hospital practitioner will argue that treatment should be targeted at the highest risk group; the public health practitioner would wish to tackle the whole population as well as those at high risk, and the primary care practitioner will take both a population-based and an individual patient approach, applying policies for cholesterol reduction across the whole practice list, and also treating individual patients (Fig. 1.7). Knowing which approach to adopt to make the most difference is no easy matter[31].

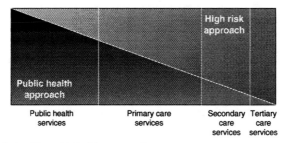

Fig. 1.7 Public health or high risk approach.

Concept 4: the hierarchy of prevention

Preventing disease is one of the key principles of public health. However, prevention does not just mean health promotion. There are many opportunities for prevention at all points of the disease pathway and at all ages of life.

One way to think of prevention is to describe it in terms of whether it is primary, secondary or tertiary.

1. **Primary prevention:** aims to promote wellbeing and to prevent the onset of disease by reducing risk factors in the population either through changes in behaviour and lifestyle, or through changes in the environment supported by appropriate public policies and health education.

2. **Secondary prevention:** aims to halt the progress of an established but possibly asymptomatic disease through early diagnosis and treatment. One example of secondary prevention is screening asymptomatic people for a disease, backed up by counselling, health education and effective treatment.

3. **Tertiary prevention:** aims to prevent disease progression and attendant suffering after a disease is clinically obvious and a diagnosis established. Tertiary prevention activities involve the care of established disease, with attempts made to restore to highest function, minimize the negative effects of disease and prevent disease-related complications.

In clinical practice, all three approaches are relevant, as demonstrated in Box 1.7.

Box 1.7 Primary, secondary and tertiary prevention of coronary heart disease

Primary prevention

Promoting physical activity through health walks for patients in the practice

Promoting healthier diets in patient consultations

Helping patients stop smoking

Secondary prevention

Screening for and management of hypertension

Screening for and management of raised cholesterol.

Tertiary prevention

Management of patients with angina

Cardiac rehabilitation

Management of people with established heart disease

Management of patients with heart failure

Treatment of acute myocardial infarction with clot-busting drugs

Table 1.2 Prevention: contributions of primary care and public health

	Primary care service	The contribution of public health to the primary care service
Primary prevention	Stop smoking services— before disease is established	Design of services for stopping smoking, and evaluation of impact
	A Walking for Health referral scheme	Wider strategy for physical activity in locality incorporates this scheme as well as others, e.g. safe play spaces
Secondary prevention	Management of hypertension detected through routine check	Monitor compliance with good practice guidelines
	Prescription of nicotine replacement	Prioritize on basis of evidence of best outcome
Tertiary prevention	Cardiac rehabilitation programme	Design and evaluate service across sectors
		Promote NHS: local authority joint working

Prevention also provides a good example of the synergy between public health and primary care in practice as shown in Table 1.2. The GP consultation offers many opportunities for prevention at all levels. Public health colleagues in PCTs can support individual input through their work with communities and health, and wider systems.

A strategy for prevention needs to combine efforts to prevent disease at these three levels. This approach is reflected in National Service Frameworks.

Concept 5: pathway of care and integrating the vertical and horizontal approaches

Successive national health strategies (http://www.dh.gov.uk/PolicyAndGuidance/ HealthAndSocialCareTopics/fs/en) set out programmes for the prevention and treatment of diseases, for example coronary heart disease. They have consistently recognized the need for a strategic approach to disease management which starts upstream with promoting and improving health as a first step (see Fig. 1.8).

This approach has underpinned the development of National Service Frameworks for the management of common diseases (Box 1.8).

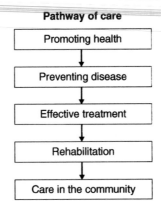

Fig. 1.8 The pathway of care.

Box 1.8 What are National Service Frameworks? (www.dh.gov.uk)

National Service Frameworks

♦ Set national standards and identify key interventions for a defined service or care group.

♦ Put in place strategies to support implementation.

♦ Establish ways to ensure progress within an agreed time scale.

♦ Form one of a range of measures to raise quality and decrease variations in service.

The rolling programme of National Service Frameworks, launched in April 1998, covers:

♦ Paediatric intensive care (1998)

♦ Mental health (September 1999)

♦ Coronary heart disease (March 2000)

♦ The national cancer plan (September 2000)

♦ Older people (March 2001)

♦ Diabetes (Standards December 2001, Delivery Strategy January 2003)

♦ Renal services—Part one, dialysis and transplantation (January 2004); Part two, chronic kidney disease, acute renal failure and end of life care (February 2005)

♦ Children, young people and maternity services (September 2004)

♦ Long-term conditions—this covers neurological conditions (March 2005)

The National Service Frameworks set national standards, and their recommendations are based on available evidence of best practice. As well as addressing prevention, they summarize effective treatment to reduce the risk of death and improve the long-term health of those who have a disease. They reflect the advice provided by National Institute for Health and Clinical Excellence (NICE; http://www.nice.org.uk) and they are used to establish the standards used in other policy documents and approaches, for example the standards in the GP contract and the standards set by the Healthcare Commission (http://www.healthcarecommission.org.uk).

The problem in adopting this approach is, however, that many people, especially as they get older, do not just have one disease but suffer multiple morbidity. So whilst logical approaches to disease management are attractive and help clarify our thinking about a strategic approach, life may not seem so simple to a clinician when dealing with a patient who not only has osteoarthritis and diabetes but also a past history of cancer and heart disease and lives in unsuitable housing with too many stairs. Integration of the vertical policy approach with the horizontal community-based approaches is one of the challenges of aligning perspectives between primary care and public health. This will be explored in the next chapter.

Summary

In this chapter we have sought to

+ *Describe the history of public health*: drawing on historical origins to illustrate the development of modern public health practice and its relationships with primary care.

+ *Trace recent policy which has shaped public health thinking*: emphasizing the shift towards public health in primary care, the importance of reducing health inequalities and the focus on local partnerships to address the determinants of health as well as the delivery of high quality patient care.

+ *Describe some key concepts which underpin the practice of public health*:

  • three domains of public health practice
  • lifecourse approach
  • balancing individual and population interventions
  • the hierarchy of prevention
  • pathways of care and integrating vertical and horizontal approaches.

In doing so we have described what we mean by a public health approach. We have considered the implications for and the relationship with primary care.

Future chapters will draw on this to develop our theme of the interdependence of public health and primary care.

References

1. Rosen G. *A History of Public Health*. New York: The Johns Hopkins University Press, 1993.
2. Ashton J. 'Past and present public health in Liverpool'. In: Griffiths S, Hunter D, ed. *Perspectives in Public Health*. Oxford: Radcliffe Medical Press, 1999; 23–33.
3. Warin JF. City of Oxford. *Annual Report of the Medical Officer of Health for the Year 1973*. Oxford: Bocardo & Church Army Press, 1973.
4. Rivett GC. *From Cradle to Grave: Fifty Years of the NHS*. London: King's Fund, 1998.
5. Department of Health. *Public Health in England*. Report of the Committee of Inquiry into the Future Development of the Public Health Function. London: Department of Health, 1988.
6. World Health Organization. *The Ottawa Charter on Health Promotion*. Ottawa: World Health Organization, 1986.
7. World Health Organization: *Declaration of Alma Ata*. Alma Ata: World Health Organization, 1978.
8. Ashton J, Seymour H. *The New Public Helath*. Milton Keynes: Open University Press, 1988.
9. World Health Organization. *The Bangkok Charter for Health Promotion in a Globalized*. Bangkok: World Health Organization, 2005.
10. Cockburn A. *Infectious Diseases: Their Evolution and Eradication*. Baltimore: Johns Hopkins Press, 1963.
11. Institute of Medicine, Committee for the Study of the Future of Public Health. *The Future of Public Health*. Washington, DC: National Academy Press, 1988.
12. World Health Organization. *The World Health Report 2002—Reducing Risks, Promoting Healthy Life*. Geneva: World Health Organization, 2002.
13. Strong K, Mathers CD, Leeder S, Beaglehole R. Preventing chronic disease: how many lives can we save? *Lancet* 2005; 366: 1578–1582.
14. Department of Health. *Choosing Health: Making Healthy Choices Easier*. London: Department of Health, 2004.
15. Starfield B. Primary and specialty care interfaces: the imperative of disease continuity. *British Journal of General Practice* 2003; 53: 723–7229.
16. Department of Health. *Shifting the Balance of Power in England*. London: Department of Health, 2001.
17. Thorpe A. 'Networks: supporting public health'. In: Griffiths S, Hunter DJ, ed. *New Perspectives in Public Health*. Oxford: Radcliffe Publishing, 2006; 338–347.
18. Redgrave P. 'Making joint DPH posts work'. In: Griffiths S, Hunter D, ed. *New Perspectives in Public Health*. Oxford: Radcliffe Publishing, 2006; 224–229.
19. Drinkwater C. 'Getting fully engaged with communities'. In: Griffiths S, Hunter D, ed. *New Perspectives in Public Health*. Oxford: Radcliffe Press, 2006; 115–121.
20. Department of Health. *Saving Lives: Our Healthier Nation* London: The Stationery Office, 1999.

21. Black D, Morris J, Smith C, Townsend P. *Inequalities in Health: Report of a Research Working Group*. London: Department of Health and Social Security, 1980.

22. Acheson D. *Independent Inquiry into Inequalities in Health*. London: The Stationery Office, 1998.

23. Department of Health. *Tackling Health Inequalities: Summary of the 2002 Cross Cutting Review*. London: Department of Health, 2002

24. Department of Health. *Tackling Health Inequalities: A Programme for Action*. London: Department of Health. 2003

25. Judge K, Platt S, Costongs C, Jurczak K. *Health Inequalities: A Challenge for Europe*. An independent report commissioned by and published under the auspices of the UK Presidency October 2005.

26. HM Treasury. *Securing Our Future, Taking a Long Term View*. London: HM Treasury, 2002.

27. HM Treasury. *Securing Good Health for the Whole Population*. London, HM Treasury, 2004.

28. Wanless D. The challenges for public health. In: Griffiths S, Hunter D, ed. *New Perspectives in Public Health*. Oxford: Radcliffe Press, 2006; 11–18.

29. Griffiths S, Jewell T, Donnelly P. Public health in practice: the three domains of public health. *Public Health* 2005; 119: 907–913.

30. Smith DG, Lynch JW. Socioeconomic differentials. In: Kuh D, Ben-Shlomo Y, ed. *A Lifecourse Approach to Chronic Disease Epidemiology*, Vol. 2. Oxford: Oxford University Press, 2003.

31. Lynch J, Harper S. Preventing coronary heart disease. *British Medical Journal* 2006; 332: 617–618.

2

Organization of primary care

This chapter reviews the current structure and organization of primary care. The last decade has been a period of continuing change. We consider the recent evolution of a 'primary care-led NHS' and how this has affected practice at ground level. Policy developments are considered from a public health perspective. We define those public health interventions that primary care professionals provide. Finally, we examine future ways of working and the opportunities they present to advance public health goals.

Historical origins

The profession of general practice derived over the course of the nineteenth century from the trade of apothecaries who dispensed medicines. In the growing industrial cities where GPs relied on patients' fees, nobody was seen in the out-patient clinics of charitable hospitals unless referred by a GP. This coverage was the origin of the first of three fundamental principles of general practice in the UK, that of referral, whereby GPs became the 'gatekeepers' to secondary care[1].

The second principle concerns non-specialization, since most scientific advances and medical care took place in hospitals. The evolution of the 'expert generalist', able to coordinate the management of patients from the centre of a web of health professionals, is seen as a source of the NHS's efficiency. By the beginning of the twentieth century, GPs were increasingly being paid an insurance fee by patients as members of 'sick clubs'. These foreran the National Insurance Act in 1911, which covered wage earners. This was extended to the whole population with the creation of the NHS in 1948, which provided the basis of the third principle: that of capitation and a fee for everyone on a registered list of patients.

International comparisons of the extent to which health systems are primary care orientated suggests that those countries with more generalist family doctors acting as gatekeepers with registered lists are more likely to have better health outcomes as well as lower costs and greater satisfaction[2]. The relative efficiency of the NHS has long been attributed in large measure to general practice controlling access to expensive specialist services. The NHS provides what by international standards is an equitable system of health care, still for the most part free at the point of use. However, these three key principles are increasingly seen as constraining. Referral arrangements are now seen as monopolistic and restrictive. Many of this government's health policies have been designed to increase access to care through other routes. The generalist is under threat. How can any single health professional stay abreast of advances in all branches of medical science? Indeed, some question whether qualifications in 'general practice' can still be offered with academic integrity. The personal list coupled with doctors' sense of 'womb-to-tomb', round-the-clock responsibility in the traditions of Dr Finlay has provided the bedrock of family practice for generations, but is now seen as paternalistic.

The second half of the old century witnessed the continuous rise of general practice. The 1966 Family Doctors' Charter introduced financial incentives for the employment of practice nurses and administrative staff, heralding an expansion in practice-based teams. Over much of the same period following the 1974 reorganization of the NHS, the influence of public health doctors declined. By the early 1990s, the term 'general practice' could legitimately be applied not just to the profession and its clinical disciplines, but to its services, staff, buildings and structures as well. However, the tripartite division between hospital, community and family practitioner services had changed little since 1948. Combined with the independent contractor status of GPs, this structure contributed to a service criticized as poorly coordinated, unresponsive and of varying quality.

A primary-care centred NHS?

The reforms introduced by the Conservative government in 1990 concentrated on controlling cost and quality through the introduction of an internal market[3]. A central policy instrument was fundholding, which capitalized on GPs' intimate knowledge of local services, and their financial entrepreneurialism. GPs were best placed, if not best equipped, to act as advocates for their patients. However, their very patient responsiveness sometimes brought them into conflict with public health directors where patient demand rather than assessed need appeared to distort their spending priorities. For example, many fundholders invested in counselling services at a time when public health directors were seeking more money for care of severe mental illness.

Although the proponents of GP fundholding claimed great benefits from the scheme, the evidence to support these claims was equivocal[4]. Fundholding was ultimately rejected for several reasons. It was bureaucratic, involving high transaction costs. It was perceived as unfair; (successful) fundholders generated inequities in access to care (two-tierism). Above all, the internal market failed to deliver anticipated efficiency gains. Yet it did entrench political support for widening the involvement of GPs in resource allocation and it empowered those same practitioners with a new sense of their political potency.

Hence, New Labour's first White Paper formally announced the demise of GP fundholding and the internal market[5]. It tackled the need to ensure quality through clinical governance (see below) and accountability to local communities. Crucially for champions of public health, it renewed an ideological commitment to equity in access and care provision. Of fundamental importance was the move to loosen the restrictions of the old tripartite structure by moving towards unified budgets for general and specialist services. The major structural change introduced to deliver these policy goals was the formation of Primary Care Trusts (PCTs).

PCTs were saddled with heavy expectations and, predictably, moved at different speeds. While they made some progress in developing and integrating primary and community care, their commissioning and health improvement functions remain immature (see below)[6]. They lacked managerial capacity to deliver the local changes their constituents demand, let alone ever-mounting responsibilities as defined centrally. Many practitioners have been disengaged from the work of PCTs—a major impediment to their success.

How does primary care deliver public health?

The key roles of general practice have been eloquently described as 'firstly, to serve as interpreter and guardian at the interface between illness and disease and, secondly, to serve as a witness to the patient's experience of illness and disease'[7]. This view originates from the psychodynamic school of GP writers and researchers who so influenced the profession in the 1960s[8]. If general practice is not primarily about disease prevention, there has nevertheless always been a strong public health tradition within the discipline[9].

With the decline in infectious diseases and ageing of the population, an increasing proportion of the workload in general practice deals with the consequences of chronic disease. This has required the development of new services and changing systems of care. Many diseases such as diabetes that were once the exclusive preserve of hospital specialists are now managed by teams in the community. If the 1970s saw the birth of a 'New Public Health', the first years of the millennium have seen the emergence of a 'New Primary Care' at least in the UK (Box 2.1). How each of these five elements contributes to public health is considered below.

> ## Box 2.1 Elements of today's primary care
>
> ◆ Self-care
> ◆ First contact care
> ◆ Chronic disease management
> ◆ Health promotion in primary care
> ◆ Primary care management

Self-care and knowledge management

Fewer than one in ten of ailments experienced are brought into contact with the formal system of health care. Most are self-managed using whatever knowledge and support is available to the sufferer. Traditionally, medicine has been based on knowledge acquired during training and topped up from time to time from sources such as scientific journals, conferences and medical libraries. These dated quickly, but clinicians nevertheless had more knowledge than their patients who were denied access to such sources. However, 'the World Wide Web, the dominant medium of the post-modern world, has blown away the doors and walls of the locked library as efficiently as semtex'[10]. Increasingly, patients are more knowledgeable than their doctors about the management of their chronic disease. Nevertheless, they sometimes need help in making sense of the surfeit of information available.

The computer screen threatens the personal nature of the consultation, but new tools are changing clinicians from being repositories of facts to being managers of knowledge. Some clinicians are nervous of giving patients better information, and not all patients want it. However, most people want to be in charge of decisions about their health—for the default approach to be empowerment rather than paternalism. Giving patients more knowledge or a consultation style that facilitates shared decision making improves not only patient satisfaction but also clinical outcomes[11]. Indeed, as people gain access to information about risk, a higher proportion may choose not to accept the offer of screening or treatment[12].

A single electronic record will in time offer exciting opportunities to integrate information from different providers and to support more self-care from home. Creative use of the Internet to communicate with patients will be central to future clinical practice. Expert patients and carers will be the most important element in the health care workforce.

First contact care

If the bulk of first contact care is provided by friends and relatives, the next port of call has traditionally been general practice. However, there is an increasing plurality of routes through which primary care can be obtained (Fig. 2.1).

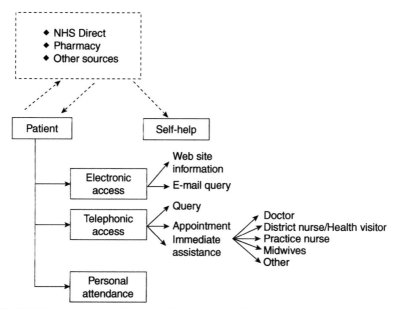

Fig. 2.1 The routes through which primary care can be obtained.

NHS Direct is a 24 hour telephone advice line staffed by specially trained nurses working from computerized algorithms. Its purpose is to provide 'easier and faster advice and information for people about health, illness and the NHS so that they are better able to care for themselves and their families'. More specific objectives for NHS Direct include the encouragement of self-care at home and reducing unnecessary use of other NHS services, i.e. management of demand. This new service formalizes 'pre-medical' levels of service but has had little impact on workloads in other parts of the health service[13].

Already sensitive to threats to their professional monopoly over first contact care, the medical profession was therefore doubly wary of the introduction of **Walk-in Centres**. Often nurse-led, these were an explicit response to the apparent success of instant access primary care facilities established by the private sector, e.g. on railway stations serving time-pressed commuters. Experience in other countries has suggested that multiple access points with poorly coordinated record keeping may result in fragmented care[14]. Questions over the cost efficiency of these new services remain. Nevertheless, they have exposed the limitations of conventional general practice in providing basic care for populations who have not, for reasons of culture or convenience, gained satisfactory access to primary care in the past.

Finally, 6 million people visit a pharmacy every day (see below). This presents major opportunities for health promotion, and traditional demarcations between the roles of doctors and pharmacists are breaking down. More than ever before, in the face of workforce shortages and mounting responsibilities, these key frontline professionals need to work together.

Chronic disease management

Numerous studies attest to the variable quality of care provided to people with chronic diseases[15]. The new GP Contract in the UK (see below) initially provided financial incentives for practices to enhance the quality of their care in 10 specific areas (Box 2.2). Much infrastructural investment is required to develop registers and call–recall systems, but the benefits in terms of public health are potentially significant. Much routine disease monitoring is undertaken by practice nurses with extended training. Disease management is becoming more complicated as pharmaceutical advances allow more care to be shifted from secondary to primary care. There is growing interest once more in North American techniques of managed care: risk stratification, targeting the heaviest consumers of care and utilization review—but little clear-cut evidence to guide policymakers[16].

Increasingly, patients who currently go to hospital are supposed to have tests and treatment in new primary care centres[17]. Consultants, who previously worked only in hospitals, will be seeing out-patients in these settings, while

---

Box 2.2 Ten chronic diseases

- Coronary heart disease
- Stroke
- Hypertension
- Hypothyroidism
- Diabetes
- Mental health
- Chronic obstructive pulmonary disease
- Asthma
- Epilepsy
- Cancer

'GPs with special interests' will be taking referrals from their colleagues in fields such as ophthalmology, orthopaedics and dermatology. The model for these is untested. Similarly, the investment in intermediate care—a bridge between hospital and home—represents a triumph of ideology over evidence[18].

Health promotion in primary care

GPs have always understood the importance of social factors such as housing, employment and education as influences on their patients' health. The registered list, which defines the practice population, provides the basis for effective health promotion programmes in primary care. Preventive activities within primary care can be divided into individual, organizational and community interventions[19–21]. **Individual** interventions take place between health professionals and patients, often classified into primary, secondary and tertiary prevention as described in Chapter 1 (Box 2.3). The public health approach to screening focuses on maximizing participation in screening rather than on informed participation. For example, current recommendations for the primary prevention of coronary heart disease in groups at high risk depend on screening through primary care and provision of risk-related advice or treatment. However, we lack evidence for the cost effectiveness of multiple risk

---

Box 2.3 Individual interventions

Primary prevention

- Health education and behavioural change, e.g. dietary, smoking cessation, exercise
- Immunization—for an ever-increasing range of infections
- Welfare benefits advice
- Community development

Secondary prevention

- Detection and management of ischaemic heart disease
- Screening, e.g. for cervical cancer, breast cancer and colon cancer

Tertiary prevention

- Chronic disease management, e.g. preventing the progression of diabetes mellitus and its complications

factor interventions delivered through primary care[22]. Presenting the uncertainties associated with the assessment and reduction of cardiovascular risk to individuals has the potential to be more cost effective than screening conducted in a traditional, public health paradigm if it results in participants who are more motivated to reduce their risks[23].

Organizational interventions are concerned with improving the management of care and access to services for disadvantaged groups. Such interventions may take place at the level of the practice or the whole health system. An example of the former might be changes to make cervical screening more accessible to certain ethnic groups by providing information in different languages and increasing the availability of female health professionals. More wide-ranging organizational changes could include the provision of nurse-led Personal Medical Services (PMS) schemes to address previously unmet needs in deprived, under-doctored locations[24].

The third category of interventions is **community**-wide. For example, in their roles as employers, users of resources, procurers, producers of waste, deployers and vendors of land, PCT have opportunities to enhance community health that have as yet been neglected by practitioners in the UK[25].

Community development has a stronger pedigree in developing countries. Every year, 530,000 women worldwide die from maternal causes, 4 million infants die in the neonatal period, and a similar number are stillborn. If the millennium development goals to reduce maternal and child mortality are to be achieved, public health programmes need to reach the poorest households. Most maternal and neonatal deaths take place at home, beyond the reach of health facilities. Evidence is growing that primary care strategies centred on community-based interventions are effective in reducing maternal and neonatal deaths in countries with high mortality rates, even if institutional approaches are necessary to reduce them further[26].

Primary care management

New public management with its emphasis on targets and objective setting has permeated all parts of the health service. One important consequence of the growth of large practice-based teams has been the differentiation of administrative functions. Today's practice manager frequently heads a sizeable team in support (see Table 8.1). Increasingly, primary care teams need to accept responsibility for auditing the health status of their patients, publicizing the results, monitoring and controlling environmentally determined disease, auditing the effectiveness of preventative programmes and evaluating the effect of medical interventions. Public health specialists still have an important role in supporting these functions.

Hitherto, practice management has operated independently of management functions elsewhere within the health service. In support of practice-based commissioning, effective financial and clinical governance, a practice will require linkages with other practices, the acute sector and the PCT. Increasingly, management functions that were once duplicated across many small units will be centralized in support of several practices (e.g. human resource management).

Other providers

Community pharmacy

Community pharmacy services have undergone significant changes in recent years. The proportion of pharmacist-owned pharmacies has dropped steadily. Over 50 per cent of pharmacists are now owned by pharmacy multiples with more than five outlets. There has been a sharp rise in the number of pharmacies located in superstores. Does this restructuring of pharmacies mean better access to services? The answer to this varies with the means of the user concerned. Superstores are accessible for those with cars but may be remote to those relying on failing public transport. The loss of a community's pharmacy with its knock-on effect across the local economy may be detrimental in many ways.

Pharmacists are taking on 'medicines management' with responsibilities for their own caseload of patients with chronic disease. More medicines are to be designated as 'pharmacy medicines', and dispensed by pharmacists without a doctor's prescription (and, in future, pharmacists will have rights for supplementary prescribing). While this may increase direct health care costs met by patients themselves, access to medicines will be improved. Electronic prescribing reduces the time it takes patients to receive their medicines, and should reduce errors and fraud. Pharmacy advice forms part of NHS Direct and one-stop primary care centres should incorporate pharmacists into a wide range of local services. Most GPs welcome the opportunity to work alongside pharmacist colleagues to better medicines management in the community. However, electronic prescriptions and e-pharmacy make it increasingly likely that many medicines will be dispensed from 'wholesale' pharmacies (remote pharmacies offering good discounts for patients with ongoing medications). This will put further pressure on the neighbourhood pharmacy business.

Finally, it is easy to underestimate the huge significance of their dispensing role for public health. For example, supplying emergency contraception over-the-counter may help reduce rates of unwanted, teenage pregnancy. Approximately 20 per cent of the NHS budget is spent on drugs, and the risks associated with inappropriate prescribing, e.g. as a cause of preventable hospital admission, are substantial. 'Polypharmacy' remains a wasteful threat to the lives of many older people. Accelerated introduction of e-pharmacy and medicines management can improve patient care. The scope for pharmacists to help improve the quality of practice prescribing is underexploited (see Box 2.4).

The new pharmacy contract provides considerable opportunities for practices to work with local pharmacist colleagues[27]. As they expand their services in support of self-care, health promotion (e.g. stop smoking services) and chronic disease monitoring (e.g. anticoagulation), coordination with local practice teams becomes of paramount importance. Close working relationships and face-to-face meetings are a necessary pre-requisite.

Box 2.4 How pharmacists can improve prescribing quality

- Aiding adherence to agreed protocols
- Giving advice/health promotion when dispensing
- Reducing waste, e.g. by identifying more cost effective prescribing options or identifying poorly compliant patients
- Closely monitoring specific groups, e.g. the frail elderly, substance misusers
- Feeding back on identified errors and drug interactions

Community dentistry

The balance of NHS and private dental care changed in the early 1990s. Discontent among dentists grew as their NHS fees were progressively reduced. In 1992/93, private work accounted for only 5 per cent of individual dentists' gross earnings; by 1996/97 this had gone up to 25 per cent. The capacity of the NHS dental service as a whole has been reduced with predictable effects: 2 million people cannot gain access to NHS dentistry.

Most of the initiatives in the government's first dental strategy were aimed at the NHS general dental services[28]. There was to be a network of at least 50 walk-in dental access centres, each seeing some 10,000 patients each year. NHS Direct provides advice on dental problems, nearest practices and dental access centres, out-of-hours services and the range of NHS treatments, including information on charges. The strategy only partially addressed the problems of people who cannot access NHS dentistry and failed to tackle the main problem facing NHS dentistry: a shift of dental work into the private sector over the last decade. In the light of later policy (see below), many observers fear that similar limitations of access will start to affect other areas of primary care.

Can primary care better meet populations' needs?

General medical services (GMS) and general practice as providers of services were left largely untouched by the internal market. The contract imposed in 1990 provided tools to increase the accountability of GPs but failed to address deep-rooted deficits in primary care and was criticized for its lack of local flexibility.

Personal Medical Services

Launched in 1997, PMS pilots fundamentally changed the relationship between government and general practice. About 40 per cent of practices now operate under PMS contracts negotiated between the provider and PCTs, supposedly addressing locally identified needs. They are subject to local targets, local budgets and local monitoring. PMS thus broke the monopoly of the independently contracted GP. Now NHS trusts, PCTs, nurses and, rarely, companies can contract to provide PMS. As a result, the number of salaried GPs employed has risen sharply. If independent contractors will not deliver local or national targets, for example in relation to national service frameworks, PCTs can now call on alternative providers. In some areas, PMS pilots have been used to increase access to services for population groups often poorly served by traditional general practice such as the homeless, refugees and people with severe mental illness. Innovative PMS practices are also supporting practice-based community development in areas of high need[24].

An important contractual extension was outlined in the NHS Improvement Plan of 2004. Alternative provider medical services (APMS) allow PCTs to commission medical services from the independent sector, voluntary sector, not for profit organizations, NHS trusts, other PCTs and foundation trusts. They can also commission services from doctors working under more traditional GMS or PMS contracts. This option aims to encourage GPs to cover areas in which it has proved difficult to recruit doctors or in which new forms of provision (some piloted in the original PMS pilots) may be needed. The ulterior objective is to improve standards and efficiency by increasing competition. Practices will need to work collaboratively if they are to compete for APMS contracts with commercial companies for whom experience of takeovers in the private sector provides an inbuilt advantage.

The alternative provider contract is one of a package of reforms introduced by the Labour government to diversify health care provision in the name of patient choice. The fear is that this complex economy will threaten continuity of care, increase the fragmentation of general practice—and its costs.

The new GP contract

Prior to 2004, the GPs' GMS contract was highly focused on the individual practitioner and failed to recognize adequately the role of the wider practice team; quality measures were sparse and crudely applied. Perverse incentives often served to reward poor quality services. The proposals for a new national contract marked an important departure.

A new funding formula is supposed to help recruitment in deprived areas that are already under-doctored. The new contract is between a PCT and a practice (rather than with an individual doctor), and services are categorized as either essential, additional or enhanced. All GPs must provide 'essential' services, envisaged as a tightly defined core, but can reduce some of their current commitments. In particular, an 'opt out' for out-of-hours care has been introduced. Conversely, practices can offer extra services for extra pay. Some of these are of particular public health significance. For example, 'additional' services include immunization, cervical screening and child health surveillance. 'Enhanced' services may tackle specific local needs such as those of substance misusers. The new Quality and Outcomes Framework covers standards to measure clinical and organizational quality as well as patients' experiences.

The new contract is changing the face of British general practice. Shifting the contract from individual practitioners to practices introduces new incentives to make greater use of non-medical staff (previously payments were linked to the existence of a GP). Patients may receive services from their own registered practice, from another practice, from staff employed by PCTs or from others such as community pharmacists. This list will increasingly include the private sector. Practices may become larger, with sub-specialization among GPs. The linkage between daytime and out-of-hours services has broken forever. The traditional family doctor will no longer be the only hub around which first contact care revolves. Continuity of care based on a long-term relationship between patient and GP is threatened.

Practice-based commissioning

Over the 7 years to 2005, the total budget of the NHS doubled, pushing total health spending up to a creditable 8.4 per cent of gross domestic product. However, despite an increase in the budget of the NHS in real terms of 7 per cent a year from 1998 to 2003, real output rose by only 3.7 per cent a year. Even after these years of plenty, strategic health authorities and PCTs were overspent. PCTs were perceived as unable to control secondary care expenditure or commission effectively. By letting GPs once again exert real influence, the government hopes that service reconfiguration can be speeded up and savings generated[29].

While there are some parallels with GP fundholding, practice-based commissioning is very different. First, practice budgets are indicative and not real, a crucial distinction if practices are to hold power over a secondary care provider-dominated NHS. Secondly, compared with the detailed departmental guidance that was always available to prospective GP fundholders, technical guidance for practice-based commissioning is limited. There is lack of clarity regarding issues such as budget setting, risk sharing between practices and PCTs, and the range of services to be commissioned. This compares with unambiguous statements about the need for practices to achieve movement towards prospective key national targets. Thirdly, the financial incentives for practices taking on these new responsibilities are limited. They will not be interested simply in managing PCTs' debts.

Will practice-based commissioning 'work'? The omens are mixed. PCTs may find it difficult to devolve commissioning responsibility to practices, especially when most of their current energies are directed at attempting to reduce overspends and break even. Secondary care may not heed the desires of practices that have only indicative budgets. Worse still following the implementation of 'Payment by Results', hospitals may indulge in supplier-induced demand as well as 'gaming'. Practices need to be persuaded that the considerable amount of effort required to bring about real change in service provision will actually bear fruit. Devolution sits uncomfortably with national target setting. The search for short-term savings may compromise public health initiatives as identified, for example, in 'Choosing Health'. For all its faults, practice-based commissioning represents the main tool this government has available for major service reconfiguration and a 'primary care led NHS'. Nevertheless, that GPs will prove efficient stewards of the NHS' resources remains largely an article of faith.

Our health, our care, our say ...

The government's new White Paper on the future of primary, community and social care again emphasizes preventive care, a greater choice of services from GPs, reduced health inequalities and better support for people who need long-term care[30]. The plan also promises more convenient access to general practices, together with an expanded range of other sources of primary care, such as Walk-in Centres. The NHS will seek new providers from the independent sector to tackle longstanding problems of poor access to health care in deprived areas. In addition, many services—including up to half of all out-patient care for some specialties—will be shifted out of hospitals and into community settings. Implementation will depend heavily on competition, strengthened commissioning and new financial incentives.

Without the counterbalance of strong commissioning, 'Payment by Results', the new financing mechanism for hospital care, together with the introduction of foundation trusts will suck resources towards hospitals. The development of substitutes for hospital care and, better still, preventive strategies to avoid the need for referral to specialists, requires strong, skilful and motivated commissioners. PCTs are in the midst of a reorganization that will reduce their effectiveness for some time to come[31].

The government's plans raise questions about the relative priority of competing policy goals[32]. In particular, what value should be given to increased access and convenience for patients, particularly when many NHS organizations are facing financial deficits? The range and volume of services provided in the community by GPs with special interests and by hospital consultants are set to increase. These service models are popular with patients, but evidence so far indicates that they increase costs for the NHS despite the government's hope that they will prove cheaper[33]. Similarly, international and UK research suggests that Walk-in Centres tend to attract a relatively affluent population and offer treatment for mainly minor illnesses[34]. The proportion of NHS resources directed towards these innovations and their cost effectiveness should be carefully monitored. Patients will be able to make more informed choices based on performance data when selecting general practices. This emphasis on greater competition among general practices may enhance responsiveness to patients' demands, but it may not prove compatible with the aim of reducing inequalities.

What were once seen as strengths of general practice within the NHS are now regarded as liabilities—the registered list (restricting choice), personal (paternalistic care) and gatekeeping (rationing). Policymakers need to be mindful of the law of unintended consequences. For example, one result of increasing access points may be discontinuous, poorly coordinated services for those most in need. Paying practitioners by results may create disincentives to practice exactly where care is already weakest. Fragmented primary care will yield poorer public health. It is a quarter of a century since Sir Donald Acheson set out his prescription to deal with the problems of primary care in the inner city[35]. Whether this government will succeed where others have failed remains to be seen. The financial and managerial climate is not altogether propitious.

References

1. Gillam S, Meads G. *Modernisation and the Future of General Practice*. London: King's Fund, 2001.
2. Starfield B. Is primary care essential? *Lancet* 1994; 344: 1129–1133.
3. Secretaries of State for Health. *Working for Patients*. Cm 555. London: HMSO, 1989.

4. Le Grand J, Mays N, Mulligan J-A, ed. *Learning from the Internal Market. A Review of the Evidence.* London: King's Fund, 1988.

5. Department of Health. *The New NHS: Modern, Dependable.* London: The Stationery Office, 1997.

6. Wilkin D, Gillam S, Leese B, ed. *The National Tracker Survey of Primary Care Groups and Trusts. Progress and Challenges 1999/2000.* London: National Primary Care Research and Development Centre/King's Fund, 2000.

7. Heath I. *The Mystery of General Practice.* London: Nuffield Provincial Hospitals Trust, 1995; 5–14.

8. Balint M. *The Doctor, His Patient and the Illness.* London: Pitman, 1964.

9. Toon P. *What is Good General Practice?* Occasional Paper 65. London, Royal College of General Practitioners, 1994.

10. Muir Gray JA. Post-modern medicine. *Lancet* 1999; 354: 1550–1552.

11. Florin D, Coulter A. Partnership in the primary care consultation. In: Gillam S, Brooks F, ed. *New Beginnings—Towards Patient and Public Involvement in Primary Health Care.* London: King's Fund, 2001; 44–59.

12. Barry MJ, Fowler FJ Jr, Mulley AG Jr, Henderson JV Jr, Wennberg JE. Patient reactions to a program designed to facilitate patient participation in treatment decisions for benign prostatic hyperplasia. *Medical Care* 1995; 33: 771–782.

13. Munro J, Nicholl J, O'Cathain A, Knowles E. *Evaluation of NHS Direct First Wave Sites.* Second interim report to the Department of Health. Sheffield: Medical Care Research Unit, University of Sheffield, 2000.

14. Salisbury C, Munro J. Walk-in centres in primary care: a review of the international literature. *British Journal of General Practice* 2003; 53: 53–59.

15. Seddon ME, Marshall MN, Campbell SM, Roland MO. Systematic review of quality of clinical care in general practice in the UK, Australia and New Zealand. *Quality in Health Care* 2001; 10: 152–158.

16. Gillam S. What can we learn about quality of care from US health maintenance organisations? *Quality in Primary Care* 2004; 12: 3–4.

17. Department of Health. *The NHS Plan: A Plan for Investment; A Plan for Reform.* London: The Stationery Office, Cm 4818-I, 2000.

18. Pencheon D. Intermediate care. *British Medical Journal* 2002; 324: 1347–1348.

19. Hulscher MEJL, Wensing M, van der Weijden T, Grol R. Interventions to implement prevention in primary care (Cochrane Review). In: *The Cochrane Library*, Issue 1. Oxford: Update Software, 2001.

20. Ashenden R, Silagy C, Weller D. A systematic review of the effectiveness of promoting lifestyle change in general practice. *Family Practice* 1997; 14: 160–175.

21. Rouse A, Adab P. Is population coronary heart disease risk screening justified? A discussion of the national service framework for coronary heart disease (standard 4). *British Journal of General Practice* 2001; 51: 834–837.

22. Ebrahim S, Davey Smith G. Multiple risk factor interventions for primary prevention of coronary heart disease (Cochrane Review). In: *The Cochrane Library*, Issue 1. Oxford: Update Software, 2001.

23. Kinmonth A-L, Marteau T. Screening for cardiovascular risk: public health imperative or matter for individual informed choice? *British Medical Journal* 2002; 325: 78–80.

24. Lewis R, Gillam S, ed. *Transforming Primary Care. Personal Medical Services in the New NHS*. London: King's Fund, 1999.

25. Coote A, ed. *Claiming The Health Dividend*. King's Fund, London, 2002.

26. Costello A, Osrin D, Manandhar D. Reducing maternal and neonatal mortality in the poorest communities. *British Medical Journal* 2004; 329: 1166–1168.

27. Department of Health. *Pharmacy in the Future—Implementing the NHS Plan: A Programme for Pharmacy in the National Health Service*. London: Department of Heath, 2000.

28. Department of Health. *NHS Dentistry: Options for Change*. London, Department of Health, 2002.

29. Neale J. Practice based commissioning. *BMJ Careers*, 2005; February 23, p. 16.

30. Secretary of State for Health. *Our Health, Our Care, Our Say: A New Direction for Community Services*. (Cm 6737). Norwich: HMSO, 2006.

31. Fulop N, Protopsaltis G, Hutchings A, King A, Allen P, Normand C, Walters R. Process and impact of mergers of NHS trusts: multicentre case study and management cost analysis. *British Medical Journal* 2002; 325: 246.

32. Lewis RQ. A new direction for NHS community services. *British Medical Journal* 2006; 332: 315–316.

33. Chapman JL, Zechel A, Carter YH, Abbott S. Systematic review of recent innovations in service provision to improve access to primary care. *British Journal of General Practice* 2004; 54: 374–381.

34. Roland M. Commentary: general practitioners with special interests—not a cheap option. *British Medical Journal* 2005; 331: 1448–1449.

35. London Health Planning Consortium. *Primary Health Care in Inner London: Report of a Study Group (Chair Donald Acheson)*. London: London Health Planning Consortium, 1981.

3

How is public health applied in primary care?

This chapter describes the public health process, which we call the public health helix. We identify eight steps in the process and describe their application in primary care. The helix puts people and their communities at its heart, influencing all its component steps. The process can be applied at any population level; neighbourhoods, primary care organizations (PCOs), or even at national and international level.

Public health is about change, and this model inevitably simplifies what is always a complex and messy process. Public health professionals need to influence policy, and stimulate environmental and systems changes at the level of PCOs. Primary care practitioners need to influence systems change at practice level including professional and individual behaviour change. Primary care and public health professionals are key players, with inter-related but complementary roles, as part of a public health system targeted at improving the health of people and their communities.

The public health process

Public health practice involves a wide range of skills, disciplines and theories. Public health encompasses action that ranges from influencing the determinants of health, such as a transport strategy, responding to outbreaks of communicable disease, to improving tertiary level hospital services such as renal replacement therapy. The approaches to improving health are complex, operating at different levels, from the national and international through to the local community and individual level. They involve action by organizations and individuals, by professionals and by the public.

The model we use to describe the public health process is shown in Fig. 3.1 as a helix, with people in their communities at its heart, influencing all elements

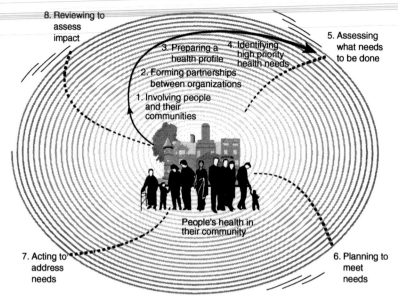

8. Reviewing to assess impact

5. Assessing what needs to be done

3. Preparing a health profile

4. Identifying high priority health needs

2. Forming partnerships between organizations

1. Involving people and their communities

People's health in their community

7. Acting to address needs

6. Planning to meet needs

Fig. 3.1 The public health helix: steps in the public health process.

of the process. We chose a helix rather than a cycle because it is continuously evolving. People's health is at the heart of the helix and health priorities are the drivers of the helical process. Invariably, this approach will involve responding to multiple health issues, and there will be multiple processes going on alongside each other at different stages of development. Although this model looks neat on paper, change processes involving large numbers of organizations and individuals are invariably messy. The model tries to reduce this complexity to a meaningful set of processes.

The model works at many different levels and different groupings. It can be used for the practice population, for neighbourhoods, for primary care organizations, for local authority populations, or at a national or global level.

There is a dynamic between policies designed nationally, such as those in White Papers described in Chapters 1 and 2, and local organizations, local practices and the public. National policy is politically derived, influenced by political ideology and responding to an amalgamation of local factors such as the causes of deaths and hospital admissions, the health impact of housing conditions or unemployment, public demands and other factors. Brought together they will produce a picture that can inform policy and practice. It is not surprising that major national health priorities resonate with local priorities.

In addition to responding to national directions, each primary care team and PCO has to be responsive to its local needs.

Other models, such as Community-oriented Primary Care[1], also address this dynamic of melding bottom-up approaches with top-down directives and are designed specifically for use at individual practice level, with a focus on team development, strategy and action on behalf of people on the practice list. This can be described as aligning the vertical approach of top-down policy with the horizontal approach of community development and responsiveness. At the practice level, there needs to be alignment between PCOs such as PCTs and the needs of the wider community, including groups not always in contact with primary care services (such as people who are homeless, or travellers) as well as the range of communities and organizations working for those communities.

Step 1. Involving people and their communities

The people have a right and a duty to participate individually and collectively in the planning and implementation of their health care.

Alma Ata Declaration 1978[2].

We unashamedly put involving people and their communities at the top of the list of activities that comprise the public health process: people and their communities must be central to the process. The people who can best understand the problems that need to be addressed are those who are experiencing them, whether those problems are concerned with housing, risk-taking behaviours, living with an illness or receiving a service. Professional staff do not have insight into all the life circumstances and illnesses that they see as part of their daily work, and in addition often make assumptions about people's needs and experiences, reflecting their own values and judgements. The only way to understand and to gain insight into what it means to live with chronic illness or with an addiction is to listen and work alongside people with the condition and involve them at every possible stage in the public health process, from prioritization through to evaluation.

Patient or citizen?

A range of terms is used to describe people who are in receipt of services, or involved in planning or policy: patients, consumers, users, people and citizens. In this book, we will use the neutral terms of person or individual where possible but will use the term patient when we are discussing users of the health service.

Involving people and the public can improve the quality of public health activities by[3,4]:

+ Ensuring needs are appropriately identified and prioritized
+ Ensuring the range of services that people need in a way that people want
+ Ensuring services are provided fairly, equitably and accountably
+ Ensuring people have the expertise to improve their health as individuals, and collectively, as a community.

There are different levels of involvement which can be summarized as follows[3].

Minimum participation

Informing, where people are passive receivers of information.

This approach has been common practice in the NHS. The leaflets in the surgery are an example. In terms of effecting change in behaviour, providing information in an unsupported way has little impact. This is discussed further in the section on managing change.

Participation

Engaging the public as consumers in order to receive information and advice from them.

This approach is used frequently in the NHS, for instance through the regular patient experience surveys, consultation on health service changes and public meetings. Patient participation groups are used by many general practices to obtain the views of their patients.

Partnership

Involving the public as partners in order to service or empower them where they have expanded roles and control.

This approach enables people to become actively engaged in order to contribute to decision making. Community development is the most advanced form of partnership, with members of the community leading the process, and involved in defining the problem and developing solutions. An example of how communities can lead and influence the shape of primary care services is shown in Box 3.1.

Step 2. Forming partnerships between organizations

The definition of public health as 'the art and science of preventing disease, prolonging life and promoting health through the organized efforts of society' demonstrates the centrality of cooperation across organizations and communities. The case studies in Chapter 5, 6 and 7 will demonstrate this. The creation of PCTs and their equivalent in other UK countries means that PCOs can work much more strongly within community partnerships.

Box 3.1 Bromley by Bow Healthy Living Centre[5]

The aim of healthy living centres[6] is to improve health through community action and to reduce inequalities in health in deprived areas. Healthy living centres attempt to address the social, environmental and economic determinants of health which require a coordinated approach from local statutory and voluntary agencies working with local communities, who lead all aspects of developing and delivering projects. Funding for healthy living centres came from the New Opportunities Fund funded by the National Lottery.

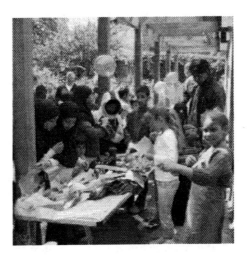

The Bromley by Bow Healthy Living Centre links health, education, arts and the environment. The community owns and manages the centre through their own development trust. The centre offers traditional GP services with the GP practices paying their rent to the trust, alongside a large range of complementary services from counselling, community education programmes, a food cooperative, complementary therapies and exercise classes. The park around the centre has been developed by the trust, and includes allotments, providing local jobs and opportunities for growing healthy food.

Bromley by Bow demonstrates how the local community can develop creative solutions for the social and environmental problems they identify, and can lead the process of community action and development that supports the most vulnerable in the community.

http://www.bbbc.org.uk

In order to determine priorities for improving health and health services, a range of organizations must be involved. The main players in health improvement in any community are usually the health service, the local authority and local voluntary groups. The health care system, local government and non-governmental organizations (NGOs) are, however, culturally and politically different; relationships between them are not always harmonious.

However, it is helpful to view these differences as providing complementary perspectives, insights and skills that are equally important. Successful partnerships will have some or all of the following attributes[3]:

- A willingness to share some of the power or control
- Ability to identify strong common goals
- Flexibility in approach and an ability to look at things from the partner's perspective
- Sharing common values, for reference when tensions or dilemma in partnership arise
- An appreciation of the skills and capabilities that other partners bring
- An environment that allows good communication, questions, challenges and risk taking.

This set of attributes demonstrates the potential dilemmas and pitfalls of working in partnership. Sharing requires the ceding of power, and this sometimes represents an almost insurmountable barrier. Goals and values take effort and time to become aligned, and time is a scarce commodity particularly in primary care. PCOs, which can speak on behalf of primary care teams, represent a very significant step forward in helping build partnerships between primary care and other sectors. Ultimately, partnerships depend upon a considerable degree of trust built over a long time.

An immediate problem faced by any partnership is how to ensure the general public as members of the community have a real say in local government. Local authorities are democratically elected, so involving local councillors on any group will increase public accountability, as long as they are able to speak and act on behalf of the rest of the local authority as responsible representatives. Every partnership needs to make considerable effort to ensure it is working with its community members and engaging local community groups as full members in the partnership.

The common ground for agencies working to improve public health is that they provide a service for the most vulnerable members of the population. This includes the elderly, children in lone parent families, teenage mothers, the mentally ill, physically disabled, problem drug users and the most deprived communities (see Table 3.1).

Table 3.1 An example of the range of agencies working with people who are problem drug users

Social services	Preventing, or intervening in, a crisis. Mobilizing community support services. Providing advice and support to carers and family. Providing benefits advice.
Mental health services	Providing treatment and care. Providing outreach services in the home. Intervening in a crisis.
Primary care organizations and primary care teams	Providing needle exchange through pharmacy. Providing treatment and care. Providing advice and support to carers and family. Providing health promotion services. Commissioning and coordinating drugs services, through leadership by public health staff.
Schools	Providing education on drugs.
Police and criminal justice system	Referring people arrested to treatment services. Tackling supply of drugs.
Housing agencies	Providing sheltered accommodation.
Citizens' Advice Bureau	Advising on finances, housing, employment.
Voluntary agencies (NGOs)	Advocating on behalf of patients and carers. Advising on finances, housing, and employment. Providing day care and employment.

This common ground enables agencies:

- To learn from each other
- To share good practice
- To complement the skills and experience of others
- To undertake joint consultation of certain communities and/or the local population.

Partnerships and cross-sectoral working are now a major plank of government policy. In response to the difficulties in joint working, the government required every local authority area to set up **Local Strategic Partnerships** (LSPs). These are bodies based on local authority boundaries, bringing together at a local level the different parts of the public, private, community and voluntary sectors. Typically they involve the following organizations:

- Local authorities (housing, planning, leisure, social services, education)
- PCTs
- Voluntary agencies

- Community groups
- Police and criminal justice services
- The business sector.

LSPs are tasked with tackling those issues, such as drug misuse, crime or homelessness, which require the involvement of several agencies to solve. The LSPs support their local authorities' Community Strategies, and Local Area Agreements (LAAs).

Box 3.2 Local Area Agreements

LAAs simplify the number of additional funding streams from central government going into an area, help join up public services more effectively and allow greater flexibility for local solutions to local circumstances.

They are agreements struck between Government, the local authority and its major delivery partners, including PCTs, in an area, working through the LSPs. They are structured around four blocks: children and young people; safer and stronger communities; healthier communities and older people; and economic development and enterprise. (Note that all of these four blocks have big implications and opportunities for public health.)

Public health issues are hardly ever solved by one agency alone. What might seem like a straightforward health service topic led by the local PCO, such as influenza immunization, requires the engagement of schools, higher education institutions, social services, private sector residential and nursing homes. Most topics are highly complex, with responsibilities for making a difference lying outside the remit of health care, but with leadership often coming from the health care community to drive through the changes needed.

Step 3. Preparing a health profile

Annual health reporting has a long tradition, starting with the Medical Officers of Health in the nineteenth century in Britain at city and county level. Annual reports are now a requirement of directors of public health, but are often undertaken at practice and neighbourhood level.

At practice and community level

There are many examples of health profiles at the level of the primary health care team. An early proponent was Julian Tudor Hart[7] who believed GPs should take responsibility for both community and clinical functions and should be accountable to the population they serve. He envisaged GPs as public health physicians, and in that role proposed they should produce annual reports[7]. Mant and Anderson similarly proposed that GPs should audit the state of health of their practice population[8] with a view to undertaking public health programmes at practice level. The approach known as Community-oriented Primary Care[9], has a health profile, or community diagnosis, as a core element. The community diagnosis requires data from a variety of sources, of which the most valuable is the qualitative knowledge about the local community acquired through years of working within it. The contribution of community nursing staff is particularly important. We describe a qualitative approach to undertaking a health profile of a practice population called participatory rapid appraisal in Chapter 4.

Health visitors and school nurses have a long tradition as public health practitioners, with their roots within the local authority departments of the Medical Officers of Health. Their public health role complements and is informed by their focus on the needs of individuals and families. With this public health responsibility they often take a lead in undertaking community health needs assessments and health profiles of the local community or their practice list[10]. Their role extends to the support of vulnerable groups in a community, and they are able to take a wider view of the health problems and needs within a community. (Sadly the services provided by health visitors and school nurses are often at times of budgetary pressures the first to be cut because they are not the subject of NHS targets.)

At Primary Care Trust level

Directors of public health are tasked with producing an annual health report, and have responsibility for analysing local statistics and reporting on the health of the PCT population[11]. Their reports consider the burden and impact of diseases and their determinants, and also quality of life issues in their community. Their aim is 'to contribute to improving the health and well-being of local populations, to reducing health inequalities, and to promoting action for better health, through measuring progress towards health targets, and planning and monitoring local programmes and services that impact on health over time[12]'. These reports provide a mechanism to highlight problems, report progress and inform local interagency action. As they address local issues, they may engage primary care teams as key contributors, and help to determine local priorities at neighbourhood level.

At national level

Health profiles are also prepared at larger population and organizational levels. For instance, the Chief Medical Officer for England produces a report[13], as do the Chief Medical Officers for Scotland, Wales and Northern Ireland, with similar aims to the report of the PCT directors of public health. Other national documents also set out the key health issues, for example cancer, that help shape national priorities. As an example, the government commissioned an independent inquiry into inequalities in health which was chaired by Sir Donald Acheson[14] (see Chapter 1).

Step 4. Identifying high priority health issues

The health profile identifies the health issues that are important to a community. Public health programmes require coordinated action, and each agency in a locality needs to be committed to the chosen priorities. In order to make an impact, local agencies can only work on a limited number of priorities.

Choosing priorities requires a process that reflects the concerns not only of primary care team staff and public health professionals but of a wide range of community stakeholders including the local population. Partnership forums such as the LSPs are set up to ensure that all views are heard; however, even through democratically elected bodies, the views of the public are very difficult to obtain. Chapter 4 explores ways that the public can be engaged in influencing priorities and the planning of services.

Decisions about priorities for planning health and health care for people and populations are made by combining three factors, evidence, resources and values (see Fig. 3.2)[15].

The first and most important step in any priority setting process is to determine the values of the community so that choices can be tested against these values.

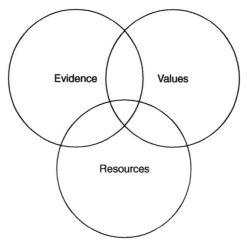

Fig. 3.2 Factors affecting decisions about groups of patients or populations.

The values of different agencies and those of the local community are likely to differ, and the process of priority setting is not straightforward as it requires the engagement and consent of all the key partners. These values or criteria are often assigned a weighting through negotiation with the partners, who then are asked to give votes or ratings to the identified key health issues. For example, some systems have selected effectiveness, equity and patient choice as the values which they use to determine their priorities and against which they can test their difficult decisions[16]. We describe this in more detail in the next chapter.

Box 3.3 Deciding on priorities for action. From the Health Visitor Practice Development Resource Pack[10]

- What is the size of population affected?
- What is the impact on health of the population affected?
- What is the effectiveness of possible interventions?
- How adequate are the existing services?
- Which priority will help meet national and PCT priorities?
- Do we have the expertise to address this problem and is training available?

Each country in the UK has set national priorities for health. The public health priorities defined by the English Department of Health are set out in Table 3.2.

National priorities help focus on what is important but result in considerable constraints on local statutory organizations, giving them little opportunity to develop local priorities unless they can be categorized under the banner of a national priority. This creates a tension with the ideal of involving local communities in determining their own priorities, and somehow the two need to be aligned. See Chapter 4 for further information on priority setting.

Step 5. Assessing what needs to be done

Having determined the high priority issues, the next step is to determine what needs to be done to address the specific health issue. Health needs assessment is sometimes used to describe the whole process of community health profiling, setting priorities, developing strategy and implementation[18], but it is also used to describe the process of analysing specific health issues. For the purpose of this book, we are using the term health needs assessment to describe the latter more circumscribed process addressing the needs for services for particular care groups or health problems.

Table 3.2 Public health priorities and targets in England[17]

	Government targets
Cardiovascular disease mortality and inequalities	Substantially reduce mortality rates by 2010 from heart disease, stroke and related diseases by at least 40 per cent in people under 75, with a 40 per cent reduction in the inequalities gap between the fifth of areas with the worst health and deprivation indicators and the population as a whole.
Cancer mortality and inequalities	Substantially reduce mortality rates by 2010 from cancer by at least 20 per cent in people under 75, with a reduction in the inequalities gap of at least 6 per cent between the fifth of areas with the worst health and deprivation indicators and the population as a whole.
Mental health	Substantially reduce mortality rates by 2010 from suicide and undetermined injury by at least 20 per cent.
Inequalities	Reduce health inequalities by 10 per cent by 2010 as measured by infant mortality and life expectancy at birth.
Smoking	Tackle the underlying determinants of health and health inequalities by reducing adult smoking rates to 21 per cent or less by 2010, with a reduction in prevalence among routine and manual groups to 26 per cent or less.
Obesity	Tackle the underlying determinants of health and health inequalities by halting the year-on-year rise in obesity among children under 11 by 2010 in the context of a broader strategy to tackle obesity in the population as a whole.
Sexual health	Tackle the underlying determinants of health and health inequalities by reducing the under-18 conception rate by 50 per cent by 2010, as part of a broader strategy to improve sexual health.

The shift to a primary care-led NHS has seen PCTs take responsibility for assessing the health needs of the population. Primary care professionals are well placed to play a role in this at a local level.

Health needs assessment takes into account the evidence of effectiveness of the service being provided to meet the needs, and is defined as 'a systematic method of identifying the unmet health and healthcare needs of a population and making recommendations for changes to meet these needs' (adapted from Wright's definition[19]).

As the role of commissioning services by GP fundholders, GP commissioning groups and health authorities (the predecessors of PCTs in England) developed, it became apparent that there was considerable duplication of effort within health authority public health departments, each working on their locally determined priorities. There is now a national system which supports local efforts, including the development of the evidence base. For example, the National Service Frameworks (described in Chapter 1) address priority conditions such as heart disease and mental health. The National Institute for Health and Clinical Excellence (NICE) prepares guidance in three areas: public health; health technologies such as medicines or surgical procedures; and clinical practice. The Healthcare Commission provides a framework for delivery.

Although these national reports provide evidence of effectiveness, local health needs assessments engaging local communities and partner organizations remains essential.

We describe the various techniques used in health needs assessment in Chapter 4 and give examples of needs assessment by primary care teams and PCOs in Chapter 6.

Step 6. Planning to meet needs

Health needs assessment identifies the evidence base for the service being addressed, determines the local communities' views about the need for change, describes existing resources and services and makes recommendations for change. The next stage is to develop a public health strategy.

A strategy for a service (such as services for drugs misuse, hypertension, sexual health) is a plan of how to get from point A to point B. Developing a strategy requires a number of processes, including addressing the challenge of managing change.

Bringing about change is complex, requiring facilitation, flexibility and leadership. It takes time, usually far longer than expected, and requires much commitment if successful implementation is to be achieved.

In Chapter 4, we describe how to develop a strategy, using the steps in Box 3.4. In preparing the strategy, it is useful to think right at the start about the issues

---

Box 3.4 Questions to ask when developing a strategy

- Where are we now?
- Where do we want to be?
- How do we involve patients and the public?
- How do we effectively engage/communicate with partners?
- How can we make change happen?
- How do we know we have done what we wanted to do?
- How do we make successful change become normal practice?

that will arise later and to document these as responses to the questions set out in Box 3.4, remembering that in real life the steps may not be sequential as some actions need to be carried out simultaneously.

To be successful, the whole process needs to be managed, with a clear project plan and a credible, respected leader, who will drive the process forward and undertake day to day coordination. Most projects will have a team to support them and commonly with public health projects these people will be drawn from across the organizations that are participating in the change process. Resources, whether in the form of people's time or money, need to be available for undertaking the development work, as well as the implementation.

Step 7. Acting to address needs

Developing or implementing a public health programme usually requires action on many fronts and, because it is directed at population groups, it almost invariably will involve a wide range of partner organizations, professional staff and the public. Action invariably means a change in the way things are done at all levels, from individual patients, practitioners or policymakers. People (whether the community or professionals) often resist change, for a variety of reasons, which can be ideological, emotional or practical. Resistance is a normal attribute, as change for many is associated with feelings of loss of control as well as genuine loss of a way of working or relationships.

One of the tasks of those taking people through change is to understand the prevailing culture of the community or organization, the barriers to change that exist, and to gain commitment to that change. Those facilitating the change need the leadership skills of advocacy, engagement, influence and negotiation, supported by evidence-based information, and a clear and targeted communications strategy. (See the section on leadership in Chapter 4.)

Implementing public health programmes requires a range of changes.

- *Policy changes*—a clear statement of the changes required, and the (evidence-based) underlying reasons.

- *Environmental changes*—to improve the environmental factors impacting on health, e.g. to improve road safety, prevent injuries, reduce industrial emissions and raise housing quality.

- *Systems changes*—to enable and sustain changes in professional practice. Systems are series of interdependent processes all working towards the same objective. For example, improving the identification and treatment of people with established cardiovascular disease requires whole system

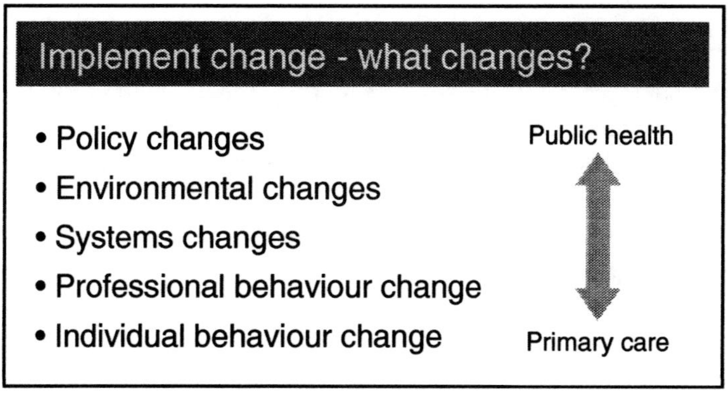

Fig. 3.3 Public health programmes: what needs to change and who changes it?

changes within the PCO and by individual practices to ensure that actions taken are logical, effective, sequential and evaluated for their impact on patients' health, with appropriate referral to specialist care.

◆ *Professional behaviour change*—most public health interventions at practice level require changes in the way practice staff work. This is part of a systems change, but there are particular tools and techniques for changing professional practice (see Chapter 4).

◆ *Individual behaviour change*—much health improvement is about enabling change in the way people act, e.g. taking more exercise, stopping smoking, adhering to treatment.

As Fig. 3.3 shows, public health practitioners work more at the policy level with organizational and community leaders, while primary care practitioners work more at the community level, supporting individual change. The tools and techniques that help achieve these changes are discussed in Chapter 4.

Step 8. Reviewing to assess impact

To be sure that all the changes made are actually making a difference for the better, and also importantly doing no harm, it is essential to evaluate their impact.

Evaluating a programme requires clear objectives with agreed clarity about standards, indicators and targets. These are defined at the strategy development stage, at which time baseline measurements are made so that progress towards targets can be measured.

What is evaluation?[20]

Evaluation is the systematic assessment of the implementation and impact of a project, programme or initiative.

It can be seen as judging the value of something by gathering information about it in a rigorous way for the purposes of making a better-informed decision. The results of evaluation activities can often be useful to others who are considering making the same changes.

One specific example of evaluation is clinical audit. Whereas evaluation tends to focus on larger scale projects or progammes, clinical audit tends to focus on specific clinical activities. Clinical audit as a process builds in a cycle of change and re-audit.

Much of the theory underpinning evaluation comes from quality improvement processes in health care, and the techniques of quality improvement are therefore used in evaluation (see Chapter 4 and 6).

It is not only health professionals who are interested in the quality of care they provide—as media interest in medical mishaps reminds us. Managers in hospitals and health authorities are charged to monitor quality as part of clinical governance (see Chapter 4). Whether as users or voters, the general population have great interest in quality of health care and may have different priorities from those of doctors. For example, they may place clear information, caring communication, and outcomes that improve activities of daily living higher up their list than technical aspects of care which may be difficult for them to assess.

However, quantitative assessment is only part of the overall evaluation. Evaluation also requires qualitative assessment of a programme through questionnaires, interviews, meetings or focus groups with patients and the public.

And the next step?

Developing a strategy is a continuous process, which is why we describe the public health process as a helix. Evaluation will show that the cycle will have resulted in an improvement in the problem or issue you have been working on, but there are more steps to take, and further links to make to other strategic cycles. Having completed the first round, you need to reassess both the public's priorities and their needs, and the national priorities (which may of course influence the importance or urgency of that assessment), and embark on the next stage of the journey.

References

1. Nutting P. *Community-oriented Primary Care: from Principles to Practice*. Albuquerque: University of New Mexico Press, 1987.

2. World Health Organization. *Declaration of Alma Ata*. International Conference on Primary Health Care, Alma Ata, USSR, 6–12 September 1978.

3. Barker J, Bullen M, de Ville J. *Reference Manual for Public Involvement*, 2nd edn. London: South Bank University, 1999.

4. Entwistle V, Hanley B. Involving consumers. In: Pencheon D, Guest C, Melzer D, Gray JAM, ed. *Oxford Handbook of Public Health Practice*. Oxford: Oxford University Press, 2001; 482–491.

5. BBC Radio 4 Beyond the Broadcast. *Changing Places: The CAN Do Culture*. 2006.

6. Department of Health. *Healthy Living Centres*. HSC 1999/008. London, NHS Executive, 1999.

7. Hart JT. *A New Kind of Doctor. The General Practitioner's Part in the Health of the Community*. London: The Merlin Press Ltd, 1988.

8. Mant D, Anderson P. Community general practitioner. *Lancet* 1985; ii: 1114–1117.

9. Gillam S, Plamping D, McClenahan J, Harries J, Epstein L. *Community-oriented Primary Care*. London: The King's Fund, 1994.

10. Department of Health. *Health Visitor Practice Development Resource Pack*. London: Department of Health, 2001.

11. Department of Health. *Improvement, Expansion and Reform: The Next 3 Years. Priorities and Planning Framework 2003–2006*. London: Department of Health. 2002.

12. Faculty of Public Health, Public Health Resource Unit, Association of Public Health Observatories. *Guidance on the Production and Content of Annual Reports for Directors of Public Health in Primary Care Trusts*. Hill A, ed. London: Faculty of Public Health, 2003.

13. Chief Medical Officer. *Health Check. Annual Report of the Chief Medical Officer 2002*. London: Department of Health, 2003.

14. Acheson D. *Independent Inquiry into Inequalities in Health*. London: Stationery Office, 1998.

15. Gray JAM. *Evidence-based Healthcare*, 2nd edn. London: Churchill Livingstone, 2001.

16. Hope T, Hicks N, Reynolds DJ, Crisp R, Griffiths S. Rationing and the Health Authority. *British Medical Journal* 1998; 317: 1607–1609.

17. Department of Health. *National Standards, Local Action: Health and Social Care Standards and Planning Framework 2005/06–2007/08*. London, Department of Health, 2004.

18. Hooper J, Longworth P. *Health Needs Assessment Workbook*. London: Health Development Agency, 2002.

19. Wright J. Assessing health needs. In: Pencheon D, Guest C, Melzer D, Gray JAM, ed. *The Oxford Handbook of Public Health Practice* 2nd edition. Oxford: Oxford University Press, 2006; 20–31.

20. NHS Modernisation Agency. *Improvement Leaders' Guide. Evaluating Improvement. General Improvement Skills*. London, Department of Health, 2005.

4

The essential public health toolkit

This chapter provides the essential public health toolkit for primary care practitioners. We use the term toolkit to cover the knowledge, skills and activities that are required to practice public health within primary care. These tools can be used to improve the health of populations at general practice and at primary care organization (PCO) levels, although we focus on those tools that can be used to make change at practice level.

A guide to this chapter

The first section **Preparing for public health action** contains the following tools:

- Epidemiology
- Knowledge: using routine data, surveys and surveillance
- Knowledge: using research through finding and appraising evidence
- Leading, influencing and collaborating with patients, the public and partners
- Prioritizing

These essential tools underpin the whole public health process and in particular they support the first four steps of the public health helix described in Chapter 3:

1. Involving people and their communities
2. Forming partnerships between organisations
3. Preparing a health profile
4. Identifying high priority issues.

The second section **Taking public health action** contains the following tools:

- Undertaking health needs assessment and health impact assessment
- Planning change
- Helping health care practitioners and people change
- Undertaking clinical audit, health equity audit and evaluation

These tools address the outer ring of the public health helix:

5. Assessing what needs to be done
6. Planning to meet health needs
7. Acting to address health needs
8. Reviewing to assess impact

Section 1: Preparing for public health action
Epidemiology as the basis of public health practice

The scientific basis of public health practice is based on epidemiology and biostatistics. Most Schools of Public Health will teach epidemiology and bio-statistics as well as behavioural sciences, environmental sciences and health systems/services/management. Study in these areas provides the knowledge base which underpins the three domains of practice. Our toolkit supports day to day practice using this knowledge base.

Epidemiology provides the foundations for the knowledge base for public health, and informs the way evidence from routine statistics and from research is analysed and presented.

> Epidemiology is defined as:
> 'the study of the distribution of disease and the determinants of disease in populations in time, place and person'

There are two broad types of studies: descriptive and experimental (or inter-ventional). Typically, descriptive epidemiology derives from routine statistics whereas experimental epidemiology is used in research settings. The main purpose of epidemiology is to describe the health of populations in a way that allows valid comparisons with other populations over time.

Epidemiology can be used:

◆ To describe the health of groups of people
◆ To explain patterns of health and disease
◆ To explain the causes of disease (their aetiology) so as to suggest means to prevent them
◆ To provide evidence for health policy and health care planning
◆ To evaluate the effectiveness and efficiency of health services and treatments[1].

This list shows why epidemiology is at the heart of the public health process.

We do not cover the science of epidemiology here as it is covered in many text books, but we give the essential epidemiological terms and definitions in Box 4.1 (see also the further reading).

Box 4.1 Epidemiological terms in common use
(NB some other terms frequently used in public health are provided in the glossary)

Case definition

A case definition specifies the criteria by which people are categorized into those with a disease or condition and those without it.

Numerator

The numerator is the number of people known to have a specific disease or condition.

Denominator

The denominator is the total number of people at risk in the population.

Odds

A ratio of the number of people who have an event to the number of people who do not have that event.

Rate

A rate is the number of people or events in a specific population (numerator) divided by the number of people at risk in the population (denominator) in a given time period. It is often given in a standard format with a time period attached, e.g. deaths per 100,000 per year.

Prevalence

The prevalence is the proportion of the population at risk who are cases.

Incidence

Incidence is the number of new cases in the population at risk in a specified period of time.

Standardized rates

The standardized rate is a method of comparing event (e.g. death, disease, admission) rates in different years, or for different subpopulations in the same year, while taking account of differences in population structure.

Standardized ratios

The ratio is of observed to expected events, multiplied conventionally by 100. Thus if levels of the event are higher in the population being studied than would be expected, the standardized ratio will be >100.

In this chapter, we signpost you to resources that provide trustworthy sources of knowledge derived from epidemiological studies, whether in the form of routine statistics or research evidence.

Knowledge: using routine data, surveys and surveillance

> Knowledge from research, from experience, and from the analysis of data is a public health resource, but at present it lies in swamps and pools and needs drainage, purification and distribution. This is a key public health task for the 21st Century.
>
> J.A. Muir Gray[2]

The assessment of health is not straightforward. There is no single measure which tells you the state of health of a population, and we need to look at a whole variety of measures from a range of different data sources to provide a comprehensive picture of health. As we have already described in Chapter 1, measures of poor health (such as mortality and disease rates) are associated with poverty and with low educational attainment. This is demonstrated in Fig. 4.1 which shows the health profile of a local authority in England with high levels of deprivation. The majority of indicators are worse than average for England. You can find information about English local authorities from the health profiles website (www.communityhealthprofiles.info).

Local authority health profiles provide information about health inequalities down to electoral ward level. There are a variety of other sources which can be useful for describing your practice population, some of which are described below.

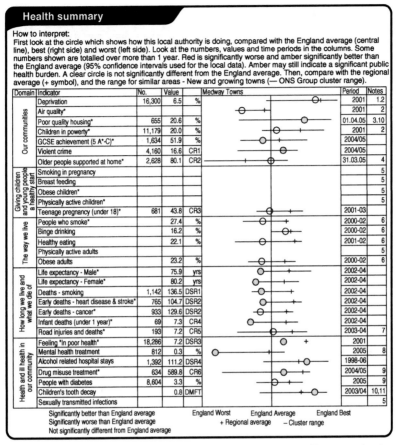

Fig. 4.1 Health summary for a local authority from the Health Profiles in England 2006 (Crown Copyright).

Data for health improvement

As with finding research evidence (see below), it is important to use trusted sources of routine information. National data sets and indicator sets are available that allow you to obtain information about the health and well-being of your local area. Some of these and other resources are listed in Box 4.2.

Public health observatories (PHOs) are another rich source of data, information and reports for your area. There are nine PHOs in England, and sister organizations in Scotland, Wales and Ireland (Ireland and Northern Ireland). They provide and signpost local and national information on a range of public health and primary care topics, and provide tools for measurement. All PHO websites

Box 4.2 Sources of health information

Local basket of health inequalities indicators

The local basket contains an initial set of 70 indicators, most at local authority area, but some at ward level. It includes measures of health status or health outcomes, measures of the determinants of health, measures of access to services and process measures.
www.lho.org.uk

Audit Commission Area Profiles

Area Profiles provide a broad picture of the quality of life and public services in a local area. The indicators, which include 45 quality of life indicators, cover themes such as community cohesion, education, environment, health and well-being, so have health relevance.
www.areaprofiles.audit-commission.gov.uk/

National Centre for Health Outcomes Development Compendium of Clinical and Health Indicators

This is an annual set of some 500 comparative indicators at national and subnational level (government office region, strategic health authority, PCO, local authority and hospital level).
nww.nchod.nhs.uk (NHS only) and www.nchod.nhs.uk (public version, but less content)

Office for National Statistics Neighbourhood Statistics

This was set up to inform Neighbourhood Renewal initiatives. It has data on a range of social, demographic, economic and health topics at ward level and below which can be displayed in a variety of ways.
www.neighbourhood.statistics.gov.uk/dissemination/

Health Poverty Index

This is a graphical summary of the situation of 'health poverty' which uses health-related data to compare populations. The indicators are presented in a variety of different formats—spider charts (the HPI chart), bar-charts, HTML tables and Excel tables.

Health Profiles by local authority

See above.
www.communityhealthprofiles.info

can be searched through a single search from one of their websites: www.apho.org.uk

Be wary of using sources where you cannot identify from the website the methods for the underpinning analysis of the indicators (and check with your local PCO's information staff or with your regional PHO if you are in any doubt, as they will help out).

Data for health care improvement in primary care

The early and comprehensive developments of computing in primary care to support care of patients has resulted in a rich source of data based on the practice list. Table 4.1 sets out the range of data available. Practice data describe the local population. These data have potential value for profiling, planning, managing and monitoring services in localities. Until recently, however, with the exception of prescribing, immunization and screening data, there has been no consistent, comparable, comprehensive national data derived from primary care. The use of data for public health purposes has therefore been limited and depended upon interested and innovative individuals at local level gathering, analysing and interpreting the data.

The introduction of the new General Medical Services contract resulted in much more data to support public health initiatives in primary care. In this new contract, all practices are paid on the basis of achieving certain quality standards through the Quality and Outcome Framework (QOF) (see Chapter 2). The framework measures achievement through clinical and other outcome indicators. The recording of lifestyle factors (e.g. on smoking, obesity) and physiological data (e.g. cholesterol, blood pressure) is required. Data from the patient records are submitted nationally for analysis in order to determine payments to the practices. The data are submitted to the Quality Management and Analysis System (QMAS) to support the calculation of general practice payments. A monthly extract from this system is created by practice and is available on the Quality Prevalence and Indicator Database (QPID)[3].

The information on QPID is available on www.ic.nhs.uk/services/qof/ and is based on general practices which have disease registers and where there are valid list size data from the 'Exeter System'. The first year of the new contract was 2004/5 and so this was the first time that disease prevalence data from primary care were available on a consistent national basis. The data can be used to create prevalence rates by practice and by PCO. The data quality depends upon the quality of recording by primary care staff, and the coding is very variable both in completeness and in accuracy. Also at present the prevalence rates are not adjusted for age and sex, unlike most other public health data sets.

Table 4.1 Data available at practice level

Prevalence of chronic illnesses (Quality and Outcome Framework)

Incidence of acute illnesses and symptoms (computer searches possible)

Contacts with GPs
 Surgery consultation rate/1000 patients/per year
 House call rate/1000
 Out-of-hours visits/1000
 Telephone advice/1000

Contacts with other members of the primary health care team
 Practice nurse
 Health visitor
 District nurse
 Others

Prescribing details
 Repeat (from computer register)
 Total prescribing figures (PACT or Scottish prescribing analysis)

Use of investigations
 Laboratory samples (bacteriology, haematology, etc.)
 Radiology
 ECGs

Out-patient referrals
 Hospital, by speciality
 Physiotherapy, chiropody, occupational therapy

Attendance rate at accident and emergency department

Hospital admissions

Health promotion and disease prevention data
 Smoking, alcohol and drug misuse, BMI data
 Immunization coverage levels (2-year-olds and 5-year-olds)
 Cervical cytology

Death register
 Cause, place of death, preventable factors

Socio-economic status
 Details of deprivation payments
 Telephone ownership percentage
 Medical records may reveal unemployment, domestic problems

Knowledge (explicit and implicit of the primary health care team)
 Health visitor: practice profile, breast feeding rates, use of other agencies
 District nurse: workload details
 Practice nurse: workload details, e.g. influenza coverage rate (note that a great deal of
           data from community nurses are forwarded to their managers without
           informing the primary health care team

Other sources
 Suggestions box

However, recording, quality and presentation of data will improve over time and will present many new opportunities to support public health programmes.

Information from patient surveys

There remains as yet disappointingly little evidence to demonstrate that the use of these tools justifies their costs in terms of improvements to quality of care. Most patients express satisfaction with the care they receive, and such surveys are notoriously insensitive.

Relationships between patients and health professionals are becoming more customer-oriented. The increasing emphasis on responsiveness to users is reflected in the terms of their new contract under which practices are required to undertake annual patient satisfaction surveys. Aspects of care that are most highly valued by patients include:

- Availability and accessibility—appointments, waiting times, physical and telephone access
- Technical competence—doctor's knowledge, skills and effectiveness
- Communication skills—providing time, exploring patients needs, listening, information giving, and sharing decisions
- Interpersonal attributes—humaneness, caring and trust
- Organization of care—continuity and the range of services available[4].

The General Practice Assessment Questionnaire (GPAQ) is one of two survey instruments that have been nationally accredited. GPAQ was modified at the National Primary Care Research and Development Centre from a questionnaire (Primary Care Assessment Survey) originally developed in Boston, Massachusetts. It has been validated in large studies here and in the USA[5]. It has already been used extensively in this country and the case study in Box 4.3 illustrates one such experience.

There are obvious pitfalls in the use of patient surveys. Leaving them to be completed in noisy waiting rooms may result in selection bias. For example, the views of young mothers (too busy), the very old (housebound) or middle-aged men (infrequent attenders) may be neglected. Small survey samples should be interpreted with care; crude attempts to compare individual staff can be misleading, not to say destructive. Random variation may explain changes taking place year on year. However, the use of tools such as GPAQ can facilitate patient involvement in their care. We await evidence that such surveys fulfil their ultimate purpose: to improve patients' experience.

Box 4.3 Case study

The Leicestershire Primary Audit Group used the GPAQ in 183 practices for 696 doctors[6]. They required at least 50 questionnaires per practitioner for statistical validity; 3981 were analysed across six scales: receptionists, access, communication, enablement, continuity and overall satisfaction with the service. Results were compared with national benchmarks and generated valuable data concerning local experiences of primary care. Overall, 88 per cent regarded services as 'good' or 'very good' though this figure fell to 59 per cent in relation to access. As in other surveys of this type, older patients tend to be happier with their service than younger ones. There were significant variations between practices, all of which found participation helpful.

Data for surveillance in health protection

Primary care provides important information on infections and health protection issues in the community. This information has several public health uses:

◆ To enable immediate public health action (e.g. identification of close contacts, administration of antibiotics, vaccination, following a case of meningococcal disease)

◆ To detect, and then control, an emerging outbreak (e.g. increasing cases of mumps, food poisoning)

◆ To monitor impact of public health interventions (e.g. tracking of vaccine-preventable diseases)

◆ To monitor impact of national public health strategies (e.g. Sexual Health Strategy, Tuberculosis Strategy).

Certain infectious diseases are 'notifiable'—which usually means that public health action will result from the notification of the case. See Chapter 7 for a list of notifiable diseases. Clinicians notify diseases on clinical grounds; microbiological confirmation is not needed in advance of the notification. The clinician suspecting the diagnosis is required to notify the proper officer of the local authority, which is usually the consultant in communicable disease control working in the local Health Protection Unit. The notification system is important so that appropriate public health investigation and action can be taken, (e.g. following a case of typhoid), but also so that diseases can be monitored, (e.g. following a case of mumps).

Certain surveillance schemes rely particularly on primary care data, see Box 4.4.

Box 4.4 Primary care data sources for surveillance

The 'COVER' scheme[7]

Cover of Vaccinations Evaluated Rapidly is a scheme which ensures that uptake of childhood vaccinations is monitored and feedback is given in a timely manner to allow the opportunity to improve coverage and to detect changes in vaccine coverage quickly. Data from local computerized child health systems for children 1, 2 and 5 years of age are submitted to the Health Protection Agency (or equivalent in other UK countries) four times a year. http://www.hpa.org.uk/infections/topics_az/vaccination/cover_intro.htm

The Royal College of General Practitioner's Sentinel Surveillance Scheme[8]

This uses data from sentinel GPs (covering a population of about 700,000 patients). This well-established scheme is perhaps best known for measuring influenza-like illness (ILI) in the community (see Fig. 4.2). When consultations for ILI monitored via this scheme reach a certain threshold, this provides one of the triggers for the Department of Health recommending the use of antivirals. In addition, GPs participating in this scheme provide patient samples for testing early in the influenza season. This enables characterization of the circulating influenza virus(es) for a particular season. In addition, the scheme has been collecting information on a wide variety of morbidity in general practice since the 1960s.

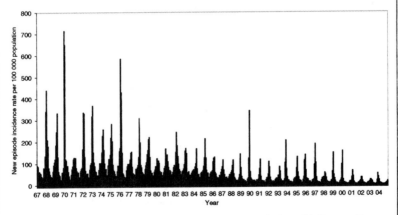

Fig. 4.2 New episode incidence rate per 100,000 population of influenza-like illness (1967–2004); mean weekly rate in 4-week periods. Data from the Royal College of General Practitioners Weekly Returns Service sentinel general practitioner network in England and Wales.

Box 4.4 Primary care data sources for surveillance *(continued)*

NHS Direct[9]

Call data to NHS Direct sites across England and Wales are used to give early warning of illness in the community. 'Key symptoms', e.g. vomiting, diarrhoea, difficulty breathing, are monitored each day and any unusual increase in symptoms is further investigated and, if warranted, public health teams are informed (see Fig. 4.3). For example, in the Buncefield explosion and subsequent fire which occurred in December 2005, NHS Direct data were used to reassure the incident control team that there had not been an acute illness in people reporting symptoms.

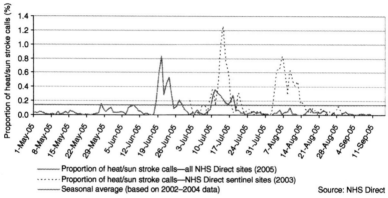

——— Proportion of heat/sun stroke calls—all NHS Direct sites (2005)
········· Proportion of heat/sun stroke calls—NHS Direct sentinel sites (2003)
——— Seasonal average (based on 2002–2004 data)   Source: NHS Direct

Fig. 4.3 Daily NHS Direct heat/stroke calls, as a proportion of total calls, for six NHS Direct sentinel sites* (summer 2003) and all NHS Direct sites combined (summer 2005); compared with the daily maximum central England temperature. *Population 19 million: North West Coast, East Midlands, West Country, Kent/Surrey/Sussex, East Anglia and South London.

Health Protection Agency and Nottingham University Division of Primary Care Collaborative National Surveillance Project

This scheme, run by the University of Nottingham in collaboration with the Health Protection Agency, using anonymized data (from the QRESEARCH database) routinely extracted from GP computer systems. It provides timely data on both morbidity and prescribing linked to morbidity. These data both provide a potential early warning of community illness on a wide population base (>3 million patients) and will enable local data to be provided (to PCT level) in the event of an influenza pandemic.

Other surveillance systems rely on data sources other than primary care, e.g. laboratory confirmation of infections and surveillance of chemical incidents.

Knowledge: using research through finding and appraising evidence

Evidence-based practice

Few people nowadays question that both policy and practice should be based where possible on high quality research evidence, but evidence-based health care is a relatively new phenomenon, really only taking hold in the mid 1990s. Now the National Institute for Health and Clinical Excellence (NICE), and other national organizations, undertake research on the effectiveness and costs of health care interventions and services to determine health care policy in the NHS. The National Service Frameworks (NSFs; see Chapter 1) also build on the evidence base to inform clinical practice. These frameworks define the care pathways, activities and outcomes for all elements of a care pathway, from prevention, primary, secondary and tertiary care through to rehabilitation and palliative care. They provide blueprints, therefore, for how care in NSF areas should be delivered in primary care. The statements in the NSFs are graded in terms of the strength of the evidence to support them.

Evidence has to be derived not only from research on what works, but also from research on cost effectiveness. The NHS does not formally use a threshold cost–benefit ratio to determine whether to invest in a drug or in other interventions. However, in practice, NICE guidance recommends that the NHS should invest in services where the cost per QALY (quality-adjusted life year) is £20,000–£30,000 or less.

As well as evidence on effectiveness and on costs, there are other factors that need to be taken into account in introducing treatments, for instance how easily new practice can be implemented, and its acceptability to patients. The decision to provide a treatment is based only partly on evidence. Experience and common sense also have a role in any decisions, as do political concerns, and the public's views are also taken into account. Take, for example, screening for prostate-specific antigen (PSA). The PSA blood test has been developed as a screening test for prostate cancer. There is insufficient evidence of its effectiveness to introduce the test routinely. However, the government has made the PSA test available on request because of strong public demand for it.

Evidence-based health care is health care that is based on the best scientific evidence rather than on opinion or anecdote. It provides a framework for ensuring that decision making, both at a policy and at a practice level, has a

Table 4.2 Best primary research design for different questions[10]

Type of question	Study design	Comment
Effectiveness	Randomized controlled trial (RCT)	The cluster RCT is used for assessing effectiveness of community-wide interventions
Aetiology	Case–control	Cohort studies also provide information on aetiology
Harm	Cohort	Case–control studies also provide information on harm
Prognosis	Inception cohort	This is a group followed-up from the start of their disorder
Diagnosis	Diagnostic test study	This requires comparison with a reference standard
Patient experience (e.g. of illness, treatment or service)	Qualitative studies	Within this there are many designs including: questionnaires, focus groups, interviews
Value for money	Economic evaluation	Cost effectiveness study or cost–benefit study (it is important that an economic evaluation takes a broad-based view of the impacts)

strong scientific foundation. Different types of research methodologies are appropriate for different clinical and public health questions, and each has its place in informing decisions (see Table 4.2). Epidemiology is the basic science behind most of these methodologies.

Randomized controlled trials (RCTs) are commonly regarded as 'gold standard' evidence. However, they are only one of several ways of looking at the effectiveness of interventions. There are sometimes ethical or practical reasons why it is not possible to use RCTs. Observational and qualitative studies can also provide valid evidence on which to base decisions at a population level. No decision making should be made on the basis of one study, and most policymakers and people developing clinical guidelines look to evidence from systematic reviews.

It is easy to forget the uniqueness of individual patient experience through the rigid application of research trials. A complementary approach to evidence-based practice is **narrative-based medicine.** This is a patient-centred approach to primary care practice that reflects the lived experience of patients. It is a form of history taking which helps the practitioner and patient make better choices through an in-depth understanding of the context within which the patient lives. This therefore allows exploration of the public health context of a patient's life[11].

Finding and appraising the evidence

Central to evidence-based practice are the skills of asking the right question, finding and appraising the evidence.

There are around 500,000 articles published in biomedical journals each year, and only a tiny percentage of these are trials or systematic reviews. For example, for the year 1 May 2003 to 31 April 2004, 3837 articles on asthma were added to the world's evidence base, but only 267 of those were trials, and 149 were systematic reviews (Muir Gray, personal communication).

Finding the evidence requires the skill of formulating a clinical or public health question and identifying the key words and phrases to search medical databases and find only high quality relevant studies.

Increasingly we now have access to high quality systematic reviews and meta-analyses of the literature. There are a variety of resources available that can support you in finding evidence, which are set out in Box 4.5. It is important to go to those sources first for trusted reviews.

Box 4.5 Sources of high quality, trusted evidence

National Library for Health

This is the library for all NHS staff, and points to high quality evidence through specialist libraries, best sources of evidence, and guidance. It should be the first port of call when looking for evidence. The National Library for Health includes Clinical Evidence and the Drug and Therapeutics Bulletin. www.library.nhs.uk/

Cochrane Library

The Cochrane Library is the output of review groups in the international Cochrane Collaboration. It prepares and maintains systematic reviews of the effects of interventions in health care to inform people providing and receiving health care, and those responsible for research, teaching, funding and administration at all levels. It is freely available to NHS staff through the National Library for Health. The Cochrane Library incorporates the Database of Abstracts of Reviews of Effects from Centre for Centre for Reviews and Dissemination at York University. http://www.nelh.nhs.uk/cochrane.asp

The Campbell Collaboration Library

This is a sister organization to the Cochrane Collaboration and it prepares and maintains systematic reviews of interventions in education, crime and

Box 4.5 Sources of high quality, trusted evidence (continued)

justice, and social welfare, which are all relevant to public health practice and policy.
http://www.campbellcollaboration.org/frontend.asp

National Institute for Health and Clinical Excellence

NICE produces guidance on promoting good health and preventing and treating ill health. It incorporated the evidence base for public health produced by the Health Development Agency. It is producing a set of guidance on public health interventions, for instance physical activity, obesity and smoking cessation.
www.nice.org.uk

Netting the Evidence

Netting the Evidence signposts to helpful organizations and useful learning resources, such as an evidence-based virtual library, software and journals.
http://www.shef.ac.uk/scharr/ir/netting/

PRODIGY

PRODIGY Knowledge is an up-to-date source of clinical knowledge that can help health care professionals and patients in managing the common conditions generally seen in primay and first contact care. PRODIGY Knowledge is practical and reliable, supporting safe and effective clinical practice.
http://www.prodiyg.nhs,uk/

SIGN

SIGN has a programme of 113 evidence-based clinical guidelines—published, in development or under review—covering a wide range of topics. Many of the SIGN guidelines relate to the NHS priority areas of cancer, cardiovascular disease and mental health.
http://www.sign.ac.uk/guidelines/index.html

Turning Research Into Practice (TRIP) Database

This resource, hosted by the Centre for Research Support in Wales, aims to support those working in primary care. The database has 8000 links covering resources at 28 different centres.
http://www.tripdatabase.com/index.html

If you cannot find the evidence you need from these sources, you will need to find and critically appraise reviews or other research studies through other bibliographic databases.

Critical appraisal requires careful reflection on the quality of the information used. Critical appraisal skills help to assess the value and trustworthiness of a research study systematically, before deciding whether to act on the evidence (see Box 4.6). Even now papers that have been published in respectable or reputable journals can have inaccurate or confusing conclusions.

It is a common temptation when reading a research paper to go straight to the results and skip the methods section as irrelevant. Yet if the study design was inappropriate, or flawed, then the results are not trustworthy.

Inevitably people interpret the same information in different ways; there is always a subjective element to this based on personal values. Judgement is key to interpreting the evidence and making a decision about applying it to your local situation. Critical appraisal of the evidence is an important part of the evidence-based public health jigsaw. More information on how to appraise scientific articles critically is set out in the references at the end of this chapter[12–15].

Box 4.6 Critical appraisal of the research literature helps readers:

- Decide how trustworthy a piece of research is (*validity*)
- Determine what it is telling us (*results*)
- Weigh up how useful and important the research will be to the clinician and to the patient (*relevance*)

The Critical Appraisal Skills Programme website has critical appraisal checklists for a range of different types of research studies. Go to http://www.phru.nhs.uk/casp/casp.htm

---

Leading, influencing and collaborating with patients, the public and partners

In our model of the public health helix, we have discussed the continual evolutionary nature of policy development and strategic implementation. We have also discussed the need to understand change (see later) at organizational and population levels. Some particular management challenges that face public health and primary care professionals in implementing good public health practice include management of change, leadership, advocacy, setting priorities, and involving patients and the public in decision making. Discussing each of these could be the subject of its own textbook, so we do not attempt to do more than reflect on these themes in this book.

Leadership

Making changes to health and health systems requires leadership, but defining what it is that leaders do can be tricky. If primary care professionals are to lead the NHS, who is needed and what should they do? Unfortunately, there is no cook book reply to this question. However, a review of some current perspectives may help understanding of what styles of leadership might be appropriate in local situations.

In their description of leadership, Pointer and Sanchez[16] highlight that:

- Leadership is a process, an action word which manifests itself in doing
- The locus of leadership is vested in an individual
- The focus of leadership is those who follow
- Leaders influence followers—their thoughts (the cognitive target); their feelings (the affective target) and their actions (behavioural target)
- Leadership is done for a purpose: to achieve goals
- Leadership is intentional not accidental.

Leadership and management are not synonymous. A manager is an individual who holds an office to which roles are attached, whereas leadership is one of the roles attached to the office of manager. Just because you are in a senior position will not make you a leader, and certainly not a powerful one. A powerful leader is one who has potential to influence.

Power comes from many sources, for example:

- *Expert power*: from information, knowledge, skills and abilities
- *Referent power*: from connections and networking
- *Coercive power*: from control of incentives
- *Charismatic power*: from one's own personality.

There are a variety of theories on leadership. One school of thought is based around the idea of charisma, with an 'ideal' set of personality characteristics which will universally be recognized as those of a leader. Theories associated with this idea include *dispositional/trait theories*. For example, from a study of US leaders in the 1980s, Bennis[17] describes leaders as: providing vision, giving meaning, promoting trust and deploying of self to the process of leading. However, different situations need different styles of leadership so a defined personality type may not be an appropriate objective. A leader does not have to be seen as a figure riding in on a white charger and providing leadership through sheer force of personality. It is increasingly common and more appropriate in health care settings to think in terms of the importance not just of the person but of the team they work with and the context they work in (contingency theories).

Modern theories have proposed two types of leadership: transactional and transformational. Transactional leadership attempts to preserve the status quo, whilst transformational leadership seeks to inspire and engage the emotions of individuals in organizations. They are distinguished by different values, goals and the nature of follower–manager relationships. Another focus of modern management highlights systems thinking, and uses concepts such as visioning, facilitation of learning and follower empowerment[18], with an emphasis on dialogue, respect and collaboration. Such leadership style requires self-awareness and an understanding of one's strengths and weaknesses and how to play to them. Increasing consideration is being given to the organizational context within which people work, and what is required of a leader in that work situation. For example, following a study of US health care workers, Klein[19] has described four key features of leadership:

- ◆ Providing strategic direction
- ◆ Monitoring team performance
- ◆ Instructing team members
- ◆ Providing hands-on assistance when required.

Such an approach leads to recommendations which are pertinent to the NHS—that it would be better to put in place necessary structures to support whoever steps into a leadership position—with well established roles and clearly defined norms—than rely on personal characteristics. Given the different expectations of leaders—and the need for leadership at a variety of levels within primary care—PCOs should encourage development of leadership potential amongst professional and managerial staff to develop their skills, their under-standing of themselves and also those of followers. PCOs can support staff and community members by providing mentoring, and opportunities for reflection and continued learning on developing leadership potential. One important role is to encourage the development of leaders from local commu-nities who can then act as local champions and advocates. Goodwin[20] also emphasizes the need for Directors of Public Health to develop their leadership skills in local communities to support the health improvement role of PCOs. His recommendations, which apply to all primary care leaders, are that they:

- ◆ Give high importance to developing and maintaining interpersonal relation-ships within and beyond organizational boundaries

- Develop and maintain extensive inter-organizational networks
- Clarify for all players the agenda for change
- Recognize the importance of creating and developing a high quality leadership team
- Build personal leadership credibility by successfully tackling issues viewed as important to local stakeholders.

Public health approaches to management

Leadership and priority setting are both practical tools for management. We do not describe management theories in detail but, since PCOs are charged with managing health care resources, we reflect briefly on some of the core principles of management, in particular the public health approach and its relevance to primary care.

Hunter has described management as having four dimensions[21]

- *Culture, principles and values of management*: management is about people, securing commitment to shared values, developing staff and achieving results
- *The structure of management*: the way organizations are set up, e.g. as bureaucracies, open systems, matrices, networks
- *Management techniques*: including communication skills, management by objectives, managing people, economics, finance, accounting, planning and marketing, project management, quality assurance
- *Settings*: buildings and organizational structures.

Understanding management requires application of knowledge of behavioural sciences as well as concepts such as power, politics and bargaining. Also, core management skills can be applied in many situations.

A common mechanism for managing the multidimensional aspects of public health practice in primary care has been the establishment of public health networks. Networks are not a new concept. We all have experience of the process of networking, be it personal, functional, social or, more recently, web-based interactions. Clinicians are very familiar with networking, particularly for providing tertiary services as well as for professional development. At its most fundamental, a network is a way of 'joining up' people with, or around, a common interest. The connections may be simple, for example a face to face, person to person connection, or a more complex and fluid matrix, involving multiple layers—like a spider's web, with different people sitting at each of the nodes where the web joins, and using many different methods of communication, with different nodes being active at different times and in different ways[22].

So-called 'new public management' is popular in health care[23]. These theories derive from the private sector and are recognizable day to day in the practice of performance management, setting standards and targets. In particular, this thinking is associated with the establishment of quasi-markets, contractual separation of purchasers from providers as an approach to cost containment in the public sector. It contrasts with traditional bureaucracies which are built on clear structures, accountabilities and chains of command.

Hunter has suggested that the market is not the best approach when considering the long term objectives of health improvement and a more appropriate style of management – public health management – can better serve multidisciplinary and community based activities at the core of primary care since it focuses on health gain and brings together public health knowledge with planning and management skills in an open multidisciplinary systems approach.

Building on this perspective we suggest that the principles of public health management in primary care reflect our basic concepts in Chapter 1 and can be summarized as:

◆ Population based
◆ Addressing health and health care
◆ Focusing on equity and addressing inequalities
◆ Engaging public, patients, professional, politicians and the corporate sector
◆ Utilizing a lifecourse approach
◆ Prioritizing prevention at all stages of disease
◆ Utilizing progammes, evidence-based frameworks and networks
◆ Engaging the community at all times.

Involving people and their communities

Most patients want to play an active role in their own healthcare. They want to know how to protect and improve their health when they are well; when they are ill they want information about the treatment options and likely outcomes; and, in addition to seeking fast effective health advice and care when they need it, most people also want to know what they can do to help themselves.

Angela Coulter, Picker Institute Europe[24]

The NHS sometimes seems more focused on the needs of its personnel than on the needs of patients, and since the early 1990s it has been trying to redress this. Putting patient preferences at the heart of the decision-making process requires expertise and time plus appropriate structures. The NHS has been slow to invest in the necessary skills, and the UK appears to be lagging behind other countries in addressing patient-centred care[24]. What is more, the structures and processes to ensure that users and the public voice are heard and acted upon have been poorly designed and implemented. The Community Health Councils, which were established in 1974 and provided a national network of independent health watchdogs, were abolished in 2003 and replaced by Patients' Forums, but these too were deemed unsuccessful and, at the time of writing, there is a proposal out for consultation on a new structure called 'local involvement networks' (LINks)[25]. These are designed to have more leverage to influence services both in hospitals and in community settings. Unless serious investment is made in these structures and in patient involvement, it is unlikely that these will be any more effective than previous models.

Patients and communities need to be involved in every step of the public health helix as described in Chapter 3. There are lots of examples of services being delivered more appropriately as a result of involving patients and communities, and indeed in the commercial world it would be unthinkable not to involve consumers in the development, delivery and evaluation of a new product or service. In Table 4.3, we set out the tasks and techniques needed for each step of the public health process. To involve patients and communities in the depth set out in this table is highly resource intensive so needs to be planned and targeted carefully. Patient involvement requires time, resources, and training and support[26]. See Box 4.7 for a case study of patient involvement.

Table 4.3 Involving people and their communities in each step of the public health process

	Tasks at PCO, community or practice level	Techniques
Step 1: Involving people and their communities	Identify what processes, structures and organizations are in place already to involve people and patients, e.g. patient panels, local authority overview and scrutiny committees, local commission for racial equality group, voluntary sector groups, patient participation groups. Set up appropriate structures. Identify skills required by professional staff and users or public representatives.	Professionals and users need to be trained to get the best out of user/community involvement. Identify who has skills in patient involvement and identify relevant local courses that can be provided for both professionals and users. When patients are on planning groups, establish remit, role, relationships and responsibilities[26] to make the best use of their involvement

Table 4.3 *(continued)* Involving people and their communities in each step of the public health process

	Tasks at PCO, community or practice level	Techniques
Step 2: Forming partnerships between organizations	In forming partnership groups, ensure that community representatives (e.g. local voluntary sector representatives, community leaders, patient participation groups) are involved	See Step 1 above.
Step 3: Preparing a health profile	The health profile is a professional assessment of the needs of the population or group. It needs to be tested with communities to establish if the findings are relevant and meaningful to the population.	Workshops and focus groups with relevant communities. Presentation to community forums, to Overview and Scrutiny Committees, local council committees.
Step 4: Identifying high priority health issues	Prioritizing needs has a professional and a public element. The criteria with which professionals set priorities are developed with communities or the public. Patients or community representatives are involved in agreeing priorities.	Workshops and focus groups with community representatives.
Step 5: Assessing what needs to be done	The views of patients or communities are essential in understanding how current services are delivered, and what could be improved.	Qualitative interview surveys of people with the condition in question or of communities (some times using rapid participatory appraisal methods). Self-completed questionnaire surveys to a random sample of patients or community members. Shadowing patients through the care pathway
Step 6: Planning to meet needs	Patients or community representatives should be on the planning group. In preparing the plans, ensure that patients/public are involved at all stages.	Workshops or focus groups Patient panels. Shadowing patients through the care pathway
Step 7: Acting to address need	Obtaining patient views on what helps is an essential component of understanding of how to help both professionals and patients change	Training for professionals Expert patients/patients as teachers working with clinicians.
Step 8: Reviewing to assess impact	Patients' experiences of services must be sought.	Patient/community surveys. Workshops or focus groups.

Methods for involving people and their communities

Patient participation groups provide a valuable forum for seeking users' views and involving them in decision making. The essence of the successful patient participation group lies in finding the right blend of critically detached but collaborative working relationship. Feedback sometimes hurts!

Though difficult to sustain in smaller practices and often reliant on the input of a dedicated few, patient participation groups are used for:

◆ Needs assessments, at the consultative stage

◆ Audit projects or the evaluation of quality of care

◆ Strategic planning within the practice

◆ Furthering involvement, for example by holding regular educational meetings

◆ Holding the practice to account, e.g. meeting to receive an annual report.

Patient panels are used to explore local people's or patients' views on local health plans. They are made up of between eight and twelve people, selected to reflect the socio-economic mix of the community. To ensure that fresh views are heard, members have fixed terms and are replaced with new people on a yearly basis. It is also possible to run a postal panel with a larger number of people sent questionnaires or phoned. This latter panel is useful for accessing the views of people who are more difficult to reach.

Panels are used to:

◆ Get people's views on plans, resource allocation and priorities

◆ Discuss complex issues.

A focus group[26] is an informal group of people who share common characteristics, who meet to discuss and share their experiences about a specific problem or experience, e.g. people with arthritis, or people who have used a walk-in service. Group membership should aim for a good mix of people in relation to the topic and should also consider other aspects including age, culture, ethnicity, gender, geography, level of disease or disability.

A focus group usually lasts between 1 and 2 hours, is facilitated and uses prepared questions and themes relating to the topic for discussion. It is helpful if an observer can support the facilitator who will be trained to analyse the discussions.

Focus groups are used:

◆ To find a wide range of experiences around specific topics with different sections of the community

◆ To find new information from participants' views.

Patient as teacher[26] is a two-stage process involving representatives from patient focus groups meeting professionals to discuss what works from their own point of view and to make recommendations for service improvement.

Stage 1: facilitated focus groups of patients, all of whom suffer from the condition, are asked questions to enable discussions on what has worked for them in managing their illness and to offer suggestions as to how the service could be improved.

Stage 2: self-selected delegates from the focus groups are identified. They are asked not to speak about their personal experiences, but to represent the views of those in their group. They then meet with nurses, allied health professions or GPs, and 'teach' them good practice from the patients' point of view and share with them the suggestions for service improvement. A plan is agreed and staff select which actions they would like to take forward.

Patients as teachers are used for:

♦ Improving the care and experience for any chronic illness where users have had a long contact with the service

♦ Education and training of clinical staff.

Patient shadowing[26] is where a patient, member of staff or volunteer accompanies the patient as they progress through the health and social care system. It is preferable that the 'shadower' does not have knowledge of the process and is comfortable asking the 'why' questions. It provides objective, observational feedback that needs to be balanced by other approaches, for example by obtaining the views of the staff providing the service.

Shadowing can be used:

♦ To map a patient process to find out what really happens on the patient's journey

♦ To monitor and measure service performance

♦ To identify training needs. It can also be used as a training and development tool to help staff understand what is important to patients.

Patient surveys The NHS survey programme requires standardized patient surveys[27,28] to be undertaken regularly in general practice. These are administered by reception staff after the patient has seen the GP or nurse, or are sent by post. The results are fed back to individual GPs and nurses as well as the practice as a whole. The survey includes communication skills of GPs and nurses, and issues such as access, availability, information giving, reception staff manner and other practice issues.

Once the GP practice has received its results, the practice staff are encouraged to invite a small group of patients to come to the practice and talk about the results. Areas in need of improvement are identified and prioritized, and solutions are planned[26].

Surveys are used

♦ To assist general practices in obtaining patient feedback for the purposes of the new GMS

♦ To help staff who want to learn with patients about how to improve quality from a patient's perspective.

Rapid participatory appraisal is a needs assessment using a mixture of both quantitative and qualitative research methods. It usually involves local people in assessing needs. This technique has been used in deprived areas in the UK[29]. Existing documentary and survey data are supplemented by interviews and observations to build up an overall picture of community life in a geographical locality.

Rapid appraisal uses selected people with knowledge of the area (residents and professionals) both to identify problems and to contribute to solutions. People are selected to represent the various groups in the area, and a key strategy is to seek out minority interests. The scientific rigour and validity of the approach depend upon the concept of 'triangulation', with data from one source being validated by checking them with data from at least two other sources.

Rapid participatory appraisal is used:

♦ To gain insight into a community's own perspectives of its main needs and to translate these findings into action.

Box 4.7 Case study: involving patients and carers in improving care for chronic obstructive pulmonary disease (COPD)

A PCT had a very high death rate from COPD and wanted to review its service for COPD in order to develop a service strategy. They invited the local self-help group to identify six patients and carers to attend the project group. An important first step was to obtain patients' and carers' views about the existing service and how it could be improved.

The project group asked GPs to identify patients and carers with COPD on their registers. Patients and carers were invited to participate as follows:

♦ Shadowing: 10 patients were followed to look at the services through their own experiences.

Box 4.7 Case study: involving patients and carers in improving care for chronic obstructive pulmonary disease (COPD) *(continued)*

- Workshops: 40 patients were identified randomly from general practice COPD registers and invited to attend workshops. The workshops were facilitated by someone skilled in working with user groups. The PCT sought views from those attending and gave them the opportunity to talk about their experiences and to ask questions.
- Focus groups: two focus groups, one with people with COPD from ethnic minority groups, whose first language was not English, and one with people who lived in the most deprived ward in the borough. These were held at community centres.

The results of these contacts were summarized by the project team and each issue generated a recommendation to feed into the plans for the service improvement.

Prioritizing

In our model of the public health helix, we have discussed the continual, evolutionary nature of policy development and strategic implementation. We have also discussed the need to understand change (see later) at organizational and population levels and to develop strategies and plans for their implementation. This brings with it a further management challenge facing public health and primary care professionals: how to set priorities.

One of the challenges of leadership is to make difficult decisions. In earlier chapters, we have discussed the need to agree priorities and how these decisions are based on a balance of values, resources and needs. It will always be necessary to make difficult choices because resources are limited. Indeed, it is said that even if the budget were continuously elastic, people's health needs and demands could still continue to utilize the resources available. The ageing population, the growth in costly new treatments and technologies, and an increasingly well informed public mean that the need to prioritize will intensify. The gap between what is demanded and what can be supplied from the public purse leads to the inevitability of rationing. What we agree to fund will depend on our values and beliefs at a variety of levels: as we treat patients, as we make local policy decisions for our PCO and as we respond to the policy initiatives of central government.

One example of the difficult local choices we make is given in Box 4.8.

Box 4.8 Example of competing demands for limited funding

At the year end, there was an additional £100,000 available for commissioning. The hospital identified three competing areas for the resource available:

♦ The waiting list for cataract operations. One cataract operation costs £715. Investment here would mean that 140 operations could be done, which would improve the vision of that number of older people, enabling them to live independently in the community.

♦ Adults waiting for cochlear implant operations. Investment here would mean that four hard-of-hearing or deaf adults could be helped to hear at a cost of £25,000 per implant with maintenance.

♦ Dementia. Twenty patients with dementia could attend the memory clinic and be given the drug donepezil. Thirty per cent of those taking the drug are thought to benefit, with variable improvements in their quality of life.

Which would you choose?

Source: *OUP Handbook of Public Health*

The issues we face when making decisions about priorities are further illustrated by the now famous case of Child B[30] which highlighted the different levels at which decisions were needed and responsibilities for them shared.

These questions in Box 4.9 can be applied to any discussion about setting priorities.

Box 4.9 Sharing responsibility for decision making

When considering whether or not Child B[30] should receive the experimental chemotherapy her father so desperately wanted for her but the local clinicians and health authority refused to provide, the following questions needed to be answered

Government:	what is the policy framework?
Health system:	what are the level of services?
Clinicians:	which treatments for which patients?
Corporate sector:	what is their social responsibility?
Public:	what are the priorities for themselves, their families, their communities?

In the *Oxford Handbook of Public Health Practice*, we describe the process of prioritization in a local context[31]. We will not go into great detail here, but in that chapter we address the tendency for inequitable, irrational decision making by constructing an ethical framework. The core values of the framework are effectiveness, equity and patient choice. Rationing decisions can be made with reference to these values, and clinicians and the public are key players in the process. However, Box 4.10 gives some of the dilemmas that are inevitably faced:

Box 4.10 Dilemmas		
Central priorities	←→	Local freedoms
Individual	←→	Population needs
Prevention (**long-term benefit**)	←→	Treatment (**short-term gain**)
Innovation	←→	Custom and practice
Professional	←→	Managerial perspectives
Patient preference	←→	Professional opinion
Providing a well tried treatment	←→	Engaging in research

To help deal with these difficulties, it is essential that procedural justice underpins an open and transparent process in which the public, professions, politicians and management all participate. There needs to be open debate about such decision-making frameworks acknowledging that trade-offs have to be made and that no solutions are perfect[20].

Section 2: Taking Public Health Action

Undertaking health needs assessment and health impact assessment

Doing a health needs asessment

Health needs assessment is a systematic method of identifying unmet health and health care needs of a population and making changes to meet these unmet needs[32]. The term describes the approaches to understanding the needs of a local population. Health needs are those needs that can *benefit from a service or intervention along the pathway of care* (health protection, health education, disease prevention, diagnosis, treatment, rehabilitation, terminal care). There are three elements to a needs assessment as follows:

- Identifying what services are available in the population
- Understanding the size of the problem in the population
- Identifying what will help that problem (what will make a service effective, efficient, equitable, appropriate, accessible and acceptable).

These three elements all have to be present for a needs assessment. No one has priority over any other (see Fig. 4.4).

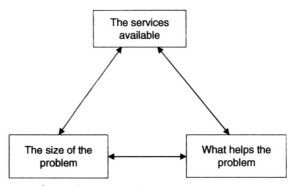

Fig. 4.4 Elements of a needs assessment.

Health needs assessment should not just be a method of measuring ill health. What matters is that something can be done to tackle that ill health. Defining health needs in terms of capacity to benefit underlines the importance of the effectiveness of health interventions and makes explicit what benefits are being pursued.

Health needs assessment tries to identify the real need rather than the expressed need or demand (see Box 4.11).

Needs assessment requires two approaches:

- *Quantitative* using epidemiology and evidence of cost effectiveness: this involves the estimation of the burden of disease or health determinant in the community, a review of the services available and the identification of the effectiveness and cost effectiveness of services.
- *Qualitative* (sometimes called corporate): this integrates the views of interested parties, e.g. the public, representative groups, professionals through surveys and focus groups, and gives a measure of demand.

Health care workers usually consider needs in terms of health care services that they can supply (normative needs). The public, however, may have a different

---

Box 4.11 Need and demand[33]

Need is often defined as the capacity to benefit. If health needs are to be identified, then an effective intervention should be available to meet these needs and improve health. There will be no benefit from an intervention if it is not effective or if there are no resources available.

Need can be described as:

Felt needs (also called wants): what people consider and/or say they need

Expressed needs (also called demand): needs expressed by action, e.g. visiting a doctor

Normative needs: what health professionals define as need.

---

view of what they are seeking from a service (demand). Health needs incorporate the wider social and environmental determinants of health, such as deprivation, housing, diet, education and employment. Sometimes the communities' needs are sought through rapid participatory appraisal (see page 88), which is a way of seeking the communities views on what bothers them and what priorities they have for improving their health[29].

Box 4.12 sets out to the questions to be answered in a health news assessment and examples are given in Chapter 6.

Box 4.12 Questions to be answered in a formal health needs assessment project[32]

1. *What is the problem?* Identify the health problem to be addressed in the defined population.

2. *What is the size and nature of the problem?* Carry out a health status assessment for the population, covering the relevant areas of ill health and/or potential health gain.

3. *What are the current services?* Identify the existing services and interventions being delivered, including, where relevant, the service targeting, quality, effectiveness and efficiency.

4. *What do patients, professionals and other stakeholders want?* Consult with a wide range of interest.

5. *What are the most appropriate and cost effective solutions?* Identify interventions by reviewing the scientific knowledge. Find and appraise.

Box 4.12 Questions to be answered in a formal health needs assessment project *(continued)*

6. *What are the resource implications?* Choose between competing ways of meeting needs (competing interventions) and decide on competing priorities—resources are always limited.
7. *What are the recommendations and the plan for implementation?*
8. *Is assessing need likely to lead to appropriate change?* Identify expected health gains.

Doing a health impact assessment

Health impact assessment (HIA) is a technique used to assess the impact of projects (e.g. a new road construction, or a Walk-in Centre), programmes (e.g. Sure Start) or policies (e.g. a local sexual health strategy or a local housing strategy) on the health of communities. HIA is generally used to assess policies and programmes outside the NHS, emanating from local authorities, regional or national government, but affecting local people. It is also undertaken within the health care setting when, for example, planning a major new health centre development or the closure of a branch surgery. One of the key principles of HIA is an explicit focus on equity and equality as often the already disadvantaged suffer most from negative health impacts, such as problems with transport with relocation of a facility.

HIA is: 'a developing process that uses a range of methods and approaches to help identify and consider the potential—or actual—health and equity impacts of a proposal on a given population'[34]. It should not be a desk top exercise, as the views of the community affected by the project, programme or policy must be taken into account. Like health needs assessment, it therefore combines scientific quantitative and qualitative evidence with local data and stakeholders' knowledge and views. It draws on elements of project management, research and evaluation.

HIA draws attention to potential health impacts in a systematic way which can have a major influence on programme and policy proposals. The kind of health determinants that are addressed through a health impact assessment are set out in Table 4.4. Primary care is affected and involved in several ways. Practice staff may be trained in doing or supporting health impact assessment. Patients and staff will be consulted as members of the community and as

Table 4.4 Health determinants encountered in health impact assessment[35]

Categories of influences on health	Examples of specific health determinants
Personal and family environment	Family structure and functioning, primary, secondary/ adult eduation, occupation, unemployment, income, risk-taking behaviour, diet, smoking, alcohol, substance misuse, exercise, recreation, means of transportation (cycle/car ownership)
Social environment	Culture, peer pressures, discrimination, social support/ cohesion (neighbourliness, social networks/isolation), community/cultural/spiritual participation, crime
Physical environment	Air, water housing conditions, working conditions, noise, smell, view, public safety, civic design, shops (location/range/quality), communications (road/rail), land use, waste disposal, energy, local environmental features
Public services and public policy	Access to (location/disabled access/costs) and quality of primary/community/secondary health care, child care, social services, housing leisure, employment, public transport, law and order, other health-related public services, non-statutory agencies and services, equity/ democracy in public policy

stakeholders. Depending on the type of project being assessed, the access to and quality of primary care could be influenced. This is illustrated further in Chapter 5.

The National Institute for Health and Clinical Excellence's Health Impact Assessment Gateway http://www.hiagateway.org.uk/ is a useful portal to a wide range of resources on HIA.

Planning change

The process of introducing a new service or changing an existing service is a complex one. Most people will initially resist change even if the results will benefit them. The whole process of change is about helping people within an organization or a system change the way they work and interact with others in the system. The ability to plan and manage change is an essential leadership skill.

In Chapter 3, we set out the elements of a strategy, drawing on the priorities and needs of the population and defining how to put into action the changes needed to meet those needs (Table 4.5).

Table 4.5 Questions to ask when developing a strategy for implementing public health programmes

Where are we now?	Do a local needs assessment taking account of local and national strategies and local people's views.
Where do we want to be?	Be clear about aims, objectives and desired outcomes Define local standards, develop an indicator set to support these, and set targets.
How do we involve patients and the public?	Be clear about why people need to be and how they will be involved. Where possible patients and the public must be involved at all stages of the strategy. Identify barriers to change.
How do we effectively engage/communicate with partners?	Involve all those who are affected by the strategy including clinicians, managers and other staff in the NHS and in partner organizations. Identify who will support and who will oppose, and develop an approach to overcoming this opposition. Keep in touch with all involved as the work is taken forward.
How can we make change happen?	Securing change is the core of the work and needs to be addressed in the planning stage. Include a description of the actions that are required, and an assessment of the resource implications, e.g. of putting the new service into place with a clear financial plan.
How do we know we have done what we wanted to do?	Evaluate the impact to demonstrate achievement against the standards and targets through monitoring routine data and special studies, including asking the public/patients.
How do we make successful change become normal practice?	The change in practice needs to be sustained to ensure that it becomes routine, as people tend to revert to their old ways of working. This requires individuals to change the way they do things. Continuing education and appropriate management strategies as well as a good understanding of how to manage change is helpful. It may also require a change in work environment with a process of ongoing monitoring and audit with regular feedback to stop people reverting to old patterns of working.

The process of strategy development brings to bear the whole range of public health tools and skills. Much of the focus of the work will be on the process of gaining commitment from partners, patients and the public, and overcoming the barriers they perceive. The final document is only as good as the process of gaining that commitment. We give an example of planning for change in a hypertension service in Chapter 6.

Helping health care practitioners change:
The psychology of change

Fundamental to change is the management of people, and an understanding of how they will react is invaluable. Everett Rogers' classic model (Fig. 4.5) of how people take up innovation helps to understand different people's responses to change. This was based on observations on how farmers took up hybrid seed corn in Iowa. The model describes the differential rate of uptake of an innovation, in order to target promotion of the product, and labels people according to their place on the uptake curve. Rogers' original model described the 'late adopters' as 'laggards'. But this seems a pejorative term when there may be good reasons not to take up the innovation. How soon after their introduction, for example, should nurses and doctors be prescribing new, usually more expensive, inhalers for asthma?

Individuals' 'change type' may depend on the particular change they are adopting. This depends on the perceived benefits, the perceived obstacles and the motivation to make the change. People are more likely to adopt an innovation[36]:

- that provides a **relative advantage** compared with old ideas;
- that is **compatible** with the existing value system of the adopter;
- that is readily understood by the adopters (**less complexity**);
- that may be experienced on a limited basis (**more trialability**); and
- where the results of the innovation are more easily noticed by other potential adopters (**observability**).

Pharmaceutical companies use this model in their approaches to GPs. The local sales representatives know from the information they have about GPs in their area whether a GP is an early adopter. Early adopters are often opinion leaders in a community. Early on in the process of promotion they will target

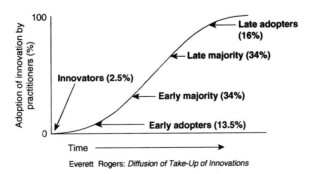

Everett Rogers: *Diffusion of Take-Up of Innovations*

Fig. 4.5 Diffusion of innovation.

those GPs with personal visits, whereas they may send the late adopters an information leaflet only, as those GPs will not consider change until more than 80 per cent of their colleagues have taken up the new product.

Any one hoping to change people's behaviour is looking for the 'tipping point'[37]. This is the point or threshold at which an idea or behaviour takes off, moving from uncommon to common. You see it in many areas of life; new technologies such as the uptake of mobile phones, fashion garments or footwear, books or TV programmes. For example, Jamie Oliver's programmes about the poor quality of school meals was the tipping point for government action. The pharmaceutical industry looks for that point for GPs prescribing their pharmaceutical product, or for customers to chose their product when buying over the counter. The change in behaviour is contagious, like infectious disease epidemics, a social epidemic. Using the model of diffusion, the tipping point comes at the point between the early adopters and the early majority. It applies equally to changing behaviour of professionals and the public.

This same technique can be used with staff going through a process of change. It is important to identify change types and opinion leaders. Knowing likely opponents is important because if they can be persuaded to support the change, they are likely to become important advocates. Understanding people's psychological reaction to change is a key to helping overcome their resistance.

Stakeholder analysis is an important part of the process of implementing change as this will help to prioritize efforts. An example of a stakeholder analysis as a simple matrix is given in Fig. 4.6. It is necessary to identify the

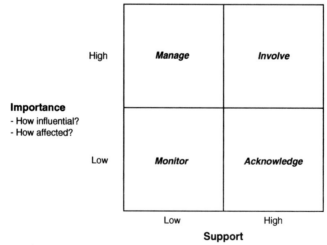

Fig. 4.6 Stakeholder mapping (*Strategy Survival Guide*[38] Crown Copyright).

most important, or key stakeholders, i.e. those who are most affected by or most capable of influencing the strategy and its implementation. Understanding how supportive each stakeholder is likely to be will then enable you to modify your approach to engaging with them[38].

- **Involve.** Stakeholders who are highly supportive and highly important should be closely involved with the work of the team.
- **Manage.** Stakeholders who are highly important but not supportive need to be closely managed with the aim of increasing their level of support. To do this, it is helpful to determine the benefits that the project can offer to them, and identify how those benefits can be sold to the stakeholder.
- **Acknowledge.** Stakeholders who are supportive but of little importance could provide a distraction and should be acknowledged but then managed accordingly.
- **Monitor.** Stakeholders who are neither supportive nor important should be monitored to ensure that their level of importance does not change, but otherwise should not distract the team.

The *Strategy Survival Guide* recommends plotting the matrix twice—once considering the degree of influence of each stakeholder, and once considering the degree to which each stakeholder is affected by the strategy. The first matrix will inform the process of achieving buy-in by stakeholders, and the second will help focus on serving the true customers of the strategy[38].

Tools and techniques for helping professionals change

Changes to systems, structures and culture are underpinned by changes in the way people within the organization behave. There is a body of knowledge about what helps professional staff change the way they work.

There are many approaches to securing change in the behaviour of health care professionals, including:

- Guidelines dissemination
- Local opinion leaders
- Clinical audit and feedback
- Educational outreach
- Continuing professional development
- Patient-mediated approaches
- Patient-specific reminders/prompts
- Financial levers/contracting.

The Cochrane Library review topic Effective Practice and Organisation of Care http://www.cochrane.org/reviews/en/topics/61.html has several systematic reviews on what works in practice and organizational change. These are summarized in Box 4.13.

Box 4.13 Evidence of effectiveness of interventions to change professional behaviour

There is good evidence to support:

- **Multifaceted interventions.** By targeting different barriers to change, these are more likely to be effective than single interventions.
- **Educational outreach.** This is generally effective in changing prescribing behaviour in North American settings. Ongoing trials will provide rigorous evidence about the effectiveness of this approach in UK settings.
- **Reminder systems.** These are generally effective for a range of behaviours.

There are mixed effects in the following:

- **Audit and feedback.** These need to be used selectively
- **Opinion leaders.** These need to be used selectively.

There is little evidence to support:

- **Passive dissemination of guidelines.** Though there is some evidence to support use of guidelines if tailored to local needs and associated with reminders.

Reviews of effectiveness have reached the conclusion that there is no magic bullet. Most interventions are effective under some circumstances; none is effective under all circumstances. A diagnostic analysis of the individual and the context must be performed before selecting a method for altering individual practitioner behaviour.

Interventions based on assessment of potential barriers are more likely to be effective.

Helping people change

Some public health programmes can impose benefits on people without them having to change (e.g. the provision of clean water). However, many preventive projects require some behaviour change on the part of the public/patient. Unless the primary health care team has the skills to assist in that behaviour change, the goals of the programme may be thwarted.

Knowledge does not always lead to 'correct' behaviour. For example, many drivers who do not wear seat belts know what happens to an unrestrained driver in an accident. Knowledge and behaviour can be out of step for many reasons (see Box 4.14).

Box 4.14 Why behaviours may persist

- Rewards of present behaviour.
- Benefits of change too long term.
- Social/peer pressure.
- Belief that change will have no effect.
- Belief that 'I cannot change'.

The present behaviour must be rewarding in some way. That reward inhibits change. For example, the smoker gets pleasure from the immediate effects of smoking; this reward is large enough to overcome the disbenefits of coughing or shortness of breath. Many risky health behaviours have no pressing immediate effects. The long-term risk of disease is too far away to motivate a change in behaviour now. The individual may find it difficult to change behaviour in a way that requires him/her to stand out from the group. If a person's work group always has lunch in the pub and the convention is that alcoholic drinks are the norm, to refrain from going to the pub or from drinking alcohol is difficult. An individual may agree that brushing one's teeth reduces dental decay and maintains gums, but may argue that 'in my case, it won't make any difference—my family have always had bad teeth'. Finally, even if all the other arguments are overcome, a person may still maintain that he/she is unable to change. 'I haven't got the will power'; 'I've tried to give up smoking three times already'.

What all this demonstrates is that telling people what is good for them is not an effective health change strategy. This section looks at more effective ways of changing behaviour.

Self-efficacy

Four pre-conditions are necessary for behaviour change to take place[39].

You must

- Want to change
- Believe you can change

◆ Believe change will have the desired effect

◆ Know how to change.

Self-efficacy is the belief in your own ability to effect change. Patients with low self-efficacy will find it hard to make changes because they lack confidence in their capacity to determine what happens to them. Self-efficacy is closely related to self-confidence and self-esteem. Where patients have low self-efficacy, it may be necessary to help them raise it. This can be done using:

◆ **Vicarious experience.** Trying to help the patient remember or recognize someone else who made the change. 'If they did it, then so can I'.

◆ **Verbal persuasion.** This can involve showing confidence in the patient ('I'm sure you can do it') or trying to help the patient recognize past successes ('If you were able to train for that new job, then you must have a lot of determination').

◆ **Successful practice.** Success breeds confidence. It is particularly important that a person with low self-efficacy does not have further experiences that will reinforce his/her poor self-image.

◆ **Achievable goals.** Overambitious goals will add to the patient's record of failure. Setting realistic, measurable goals is more likely to ensure successful practice and boost self-efficacy.

◆ **Feedback.** Physical feedback that tells you that you are doing something right increases self-efficacy (e.g. the 'feel good' factor in exercise which fuels the desire for more exercise).

Stages of behavioural change

Prochaska and DiClemente[40] have provided the best known model of behaviour change (Table 4.6). The stages can be illustrated by the example of someone giving up smoking.

Environmental influences

Environmental influences on behaviour are easily overlooked (Fig. 4.7). Antecedents are those events that trigger the behaviour, e.g. joining a group of smokers at a work break, rather than a group of non-smokers. The consequences are the outcomes of the behaviour. These will be pleasurable (the intake of smoke, the sweetness of the biscuit with the cup of tea). Hence they reinforce the antecedents. 'If I get pleasure (the sweet taste of the biscuit) when I make a cup of tea, then I will do so again'. Note that, although consequences are an outcome of behaviour, they also influence behaviour. Consequences are a form of reward. They can be tangible (e.g. allowing yourself a meal out after a week of not smoking) or intangible (e.g. praise from your family).

Table 4.6 Stages of change model[40]

Stage of change	Patient response	Your role in supporting change
Pre-contemplation	At this stage, the person is not aware that he/she has a problem. Others, though, might be pointing out the problem.	Highlighting the problem and presenting the associated risks.
Contemplation	The smoker begins to recognise that he/she has a problem. He/she thinks about the problem – is it bad enough to need action?	Providing information about what actions he/she might take and offering help.
Preparation	What action might I take? Who could help? At this stage, the smoker might discuss his/her problems with others, including ex-smokers.	Identifying 'enablers' that reinforce existing behaviour, referral to local smoking cessation service, helping set a quit date.
Action	This is when the attempt to change behaviour takes place. It can Include joining a support group; using a nicotine replacement therapy; keeping charts of progress.	Supporting the chosen course of action with encouragement and information as required, helping address enabling factors.
Maintenance	Once the smoker has reached the desired level of performance (say, abstinence), he/she has to keep to that level. This may involve special strategies for recognising a high risk situation (e.g. "When I go to the pub with the bowls team, there's always a lot of smoking") and designing strategies for dealing with them (e.g. "When the game is finished, I will remind the team that they must not let me have a cigarette even if I ask for one in the pub").	Providing non-judgmental reinforcement and support as required.
Relapse	Despite a patient's best efforts, relapses occur and patients need to be warned that this can happen. The commonest triggers of relapse are: ♦ An event that triggers a low emotional state; ♦ Unexpected, unwelcome events such as accidents, burglaries or job loss; ♦ Interpersonal problems, e.g. family rows or problems with people at work; ♦ Social pressure, especially when the pressure catches the patient unawares. (e.g. the patient goes away on business for a few days and finds that most of the business takes place in restaurants and bars.)	Accepting the relapse as normal and not as an indication of weakness on the patient's part; talking the relapse through and see what the patient can learn form it; and helping the patient re-establish short-term targets.

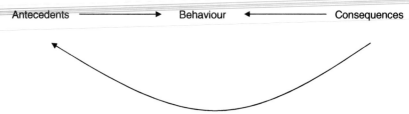

Fig. 4.7 The environmental influences on behaviour[39].

They can also be internal (e.g. feeling good about your lost 8 lbs) or external (e.g. the doctor praising you for losing 8 lbs). Early rewards in behaviour change are likely to be tangible and external. If the change is to become permanent and self-maintained, the rewards need to become intangible and internal (Table 4.7).

Behaviour change centring on individuals in the consultation is resource intensive and presents the public health practitioners with a familiar dilemma. While there is evidence in favour of various sorts of 'brief interventions' (e.g. to reduce smoking or alcohol consumption), many patients require longer term support respecting individuals' needs and confidentiality. Simple advice giving in support of grandiose public health goals is frequently ineffective, and does

Table 4.7 Overcoming environmental influences on behaviour[39]

Avoid antecedents.	For some patients, avoiding the antecedents may help to break the behaviour pattern. If a patient always smokes when going to the pub, finding another social activity—especially one where smoking is prohibited—may be the answer.
Change the antecedents.	A patient who always goes to work by car could arrange to go to work with a colleague who walks. The new cue ('go to work with colleague') triggers the behaviour 'walk'.
Establish effective consequences.	Any new behaviour pattern must have satisfying consequences, otherwise it will not be sustained. For example, someone giving up smoking may derive immediate financial benefits. Later, the rewards are likely to be intrinsic to the changed health state (e.g. feeling fitter or looking better).
Wider social and political environment.	There is plenty of evidence that raising taxes on cigarettes and alcohol help to contain demand. Governments have in the past been tardy in addressing such issues as tobacco advertising and sports sponsorship. Politicians fear being branded as anti-libertarian ('the nanny state'). However, the success of the ban on smoking in public places illustrates the extent to which the social milieu has changed—in large measure as a result of public health advocacy.

not necessarily coincide with the needs of the patient or the practitioner[41]. At times, talking about behaviour change may be detrimental to their relationship. Decontextualized health promotion interventions to either party will meet the same fate: only a few will respond. Practitioners may be painfully aware of their limited ability to counteract environmental factors such as stress, poverty, educational disadvantage and family breakdown, but to dichotomize social and psychological models of behaviour change is unhelpful. A central tenet of this book is that these models will be useful to both clinicians and public health practitioners. The GP or practice nurse is faced with the patient with presenting problems. However, the psychological expectations of the patient are not separate from the broader social circumstances that mould them. Heightened sensitivity to those social and environmental pressures is the hallmark of the compassionate clinician, and the psychological models we describe apply to the behaviour of individuals as well as within teams and organizations.

Communicating risk

Risks may be voluntary or imposed; they may be familiar or unknown, and they may be concentrated or dispersed over time. These characteristics affect the way people interpret information on risk, and the way they discount the risks over time affects their responses to them. A whole range of so-called 'fright factors' characterize those risks we fear most (Box 4.15). The common thread linking most of these factors is loss of control. BSE is terrifying because

Box 4.15 'Fright factors'—what characterizes those risks we fear most?

1. Do not involve voluntary choice
2. Cannot escape by taking personal precautions
3. Unfamiliar or novel
4. Man made rather than natural
5. Hidden and irreversible
6. Danger to children and future generations
7. Dreadful outcome
8. Poorly understood by science
9. Subject to contradictory statements
10. Cause damage to identifiable victims

it seems to strike arbitrarily, affecting young people, and results in total loss of bodily control. It remains poorly understood, as reflected in uncertain statements from government. People's interpretations of a condition and its burden also vary—for example, fear of having a stroke will mean different things to people according to their personal experience.

Risk communication is defined as the open two-way exchange of information and opinion about risk, leading to better understanding and better decisions about clinical management[42]. This definition moves away from notions that information is communicated only from clinician to patient, and that the acceptability (or not) of the risk is communicated back. The two-way exchange about information and opinion is important if decisions about treatment are to reflect the attitudes to risk of the people who will live with the outcomes.

Box 4.16 Choices depend on how risk is communicated

One hundred and forty senior managers were asked which of four cardiac rehabilitation programmes[45] they would implement. These are the data they were given about the relative effectiveness of coronary bypass surgery. During a 3-year follow-up:

Programme A reduced the rate of deaths by twenty per cent.

Programme B produced an absolute reduction in deaths of 3 per cent.

Programme C increased the rate of patient survival from 84 to 87 per cent.

Programme D meant that 31 people needed to to enter a rehabilitation programme to prevent one death.

Programme D is the number of patients who need to be treated with bypass surgery to save one life, in this instance 1 out of 31, corresponding to 3.2 per cent. The other 30 have no benefit in terms of mortality reduction. These are, of course, equivalent descriptions of one and the same outcome of an actual randomized trial in which these two treatments were compared.

You might think that in deciding which programme to fund, this informed committee would not have been influenced by the differences in presentation—but they were. The authorities saw the programme as having the greatest merit and were most willing to fund it when the benefits were expressed in terms of relative risk (Programme A). Only three out of the 140 experts realized that all four figures reflected the same clinical results.

The problems of risk language

Terms such as 'probable', 'unlikely' and 'rare' have been shown to convey elastic concepts[43]. One person's understanding of 'likely' may be a chance of 1 in 10, whereas another may think that it means a chance of 1 in 2. Any one person may also interpret the term differently in different contexts; a 'rare' outcome is a different prospect in the context of genetic or antenatal tests than, for example, in the context of antibiotic treatment for tonsillitis.

Further problems in communicating risks result from the effects of different information frames. Logically equivalent choice situations can be presented in different ways, such as advising patients about their prognosis by using either survival or mortality data[44].

We can be persuasive with information. Pharmaceutical companies use powerful techniques to present effects of their drugs to professionals. A survey of publicity of mammography for patients found that, to encourage uptake, only information on relative risk (RR) was presented. As we have seen, this format is more 'effective'[46]. Perhaps this presentational selection is justifiable in some situations to achieve the greatest public health gain, but presenting information in such a way is not consistent with truly informed decision making. The effects of different ways of presenting information are summarized in Box 4.17[47].

Box 4.17 The effects of framing and other manipulations[47]

Information on relative risk is more persuasive than absolute risk data.

'Loss' framing (e.g. the potential losses from not having a mammogram) influences screening uptake more than 'gain' framing.

Positive framing (e.g. chance of survival) is more effective than negative framing (chance of death) in persuading people to take risky options, such as treatments.

More information, and information that is more understandable to the patient, is associated with a greater wariness to take treatments or tests.

Principles for future communication of risks[47]

◆ **The information should be simple and balanced.** Comparison with 'everyday risks' with which people are familiar may help to present risk data. Information on RR should not be presented in isolation. It seems sensible to employ both absolute and relative risk formats. The former include the number needed to treat (NNT) and the number needed to harm (NNH), but these can be hard to interpret. More empirical research into the merits of these terms alone or in combination for patients is urgently required.

- Risk information relevant to individuals is more valuable than average population data[42]. For example, an individual's risk of future coronary heart disease can be calculated by using information on risk factors (such as age, hypertension, cholesterol, smoking status or diabetes) from readily available charts.

- Information must be presented clearly. Sometimes numerical data alone may suffice. The visual presentation of risk information has also been explored. Some studies suggest that many patients prefer simple bar charts to other formats such as thermometer scales, crowd figures (e.g. showing how many of 100 people are affected), survival curves or pie charts[48].

- Most patients express a strong desire for information but care is required to avoid overloading them. A major strength of general practice is that it may allow discussion of information over several consultations.

In conclusion, health professionals need to be aware of their patients' need for information, be clear what their own views are and how they may colour what they say, be practised in the use of language and the tools they use, and be versatile in their application in differing circumstances.

Risk communication: the role of the media

So far in this chapter we have described the assessment of risk in relation to an individual and their risk of disease or ill health. However, there is another perspective on risk: the role of the media. Events such as the SARS epidemic and more recently the threat of the spread of avian 'flu have heightened awareness of public health risks both in the public and in the media. Experience has taught us that good practice in communicating risk is often the first casualty during a health crisis that affects whole populations.

During the SARS epidemic in Hong Kong in 2003, the media played a key role in first alerting the public and then contributing to the panic that first ensued as the disease took hold. Rather unreasonably they led the clarion call for certainty about the nature of this mysterious disease which was affecting health care workers. Gradually, the politicians, profession and press aligned themselves to work in a more constructive partnership to inform the public as the science unfolded and the epidemic was contained.

However, the same problems also occur in communicating potential public health crises. The large-scale confusion between avian 'flu (a disease affecting birds and very few humans) and a human influenza pandemic is a topical and powerful example.

One of the lessons from the SARS experience was that it is important to have trained communicators, who are transparent in the messages they give, empathetic to the fears and concerns of media and the population, and willing to explain risk and uncertainty.

Good relationships and understanding between the media and health professionals are essential in shaping the public's attitude to risk and crisis and thus its behaviour. This is particularly important when politicians are involved. The public expects that politicians will provide protection and certainty, and that anything government oversees should thus have a zero risk. The public feels that it is unacceptable to be living with uncertainty, however unrealistic this is. It is thus very important to build trust between the media and those professions who have critical roles in dealing with the uncertainties and risks around new health situations.

In *Health in the News*, Harrabin[49] recommends more skilled presentation of health issues by experts for news features, using accessible language as key to explaining risk. Local health care workers in positions of authority in PCOs need to be able to communicate well as they will need to speak out, and may need to explain that all the answers are not known, but to do this without alarming the public. Box 4.18 sets out a list of resources that are written for patients and the public.

Box 4.18 Resources for patients: databases and websites that practitioners can refer patients to

Database of Individual Patient Experiences (http://www.dipex.org/) contains patients' experiences, including narratives of decision pathways.
UK National Library for Health (http://www.library.nhs.uk) includes different levels of information for patients.
NHS Direct On-Line http://www.nhsdirect.nhs.uk/ is a website providing information and advice on illness and well being.
Health Crossroads (http://www.healthcrossroads.com) audio overviews for over 70 decisions (or crossroads) in different conditions including breast cancer, benign uterine conditions (such as fibroids), prostate disease, coronary artery disease and back pain.

Advocacy

One of the traditional and enduring roles of public health is to champion the cause of disadvantaged groups in society. The underlying principle of advocacy is to raise awareness of critical public health issues and mobilize communities and resources to promote better health. This can either be done as an individual, for example writing a letter to support a patient get better housing, or at organizational level, for example through discussions between practice or PCT and the local council to improve the play space for children on the local estate. Examples of the levels of advocacy are given in Table 4.8.

The process of advocacy uses data strategically, identifies and works with allies, deals with the opposition, works closely with the relevant community and uses the media strategically. Successful desired outcomes of advocacy are patient empowerment, less health-damaging behaviour, changes in policy, better services, better health and a better society. In addition to the tools of health education, epidemiological analysis and promoting community participation, social marketing is becoming an increasingly popular technique to use.

Table 4.8 Examples of different levels of advocacy

Area	Actors
Institutional	National government global agencies e.g. WHO
Organizational	National: NGOs, e.g. Action on Smoking and Health, special interest groups Local: practice, PCT, local authority
Community based	Grass roots, local stakeholders, patients group
Professional	Technical organizations, e.g. trade unions, educational bodies, e.g. Royal Colleges
Individual	Highly motivated individuals, either staff, or patients or their carers

Social marketing

Recent government policy documents such as 'Choosing Health'[50] and 'Our Health, Our Care, Our Say'[51] have focused on the shift away from a paternalistic state to a greater emphasis on individual choice. Part of the thinking behind this approach has been that in the face of obvious failures to control modern epidemics such as obesity, new approaches are needed. One such new approach is social marketing, an approach to promoting health which draws heavily on the experience of the commercial sector. As an approach, it focuses on individuals as consumers for whom health is a good, something they wish to invest in.

A definition of health-related social marketing[52].
A systematic process using marketing techniques and approaches to achieve behavioural goals, relevant to improving health and well-being.

The features of social marketing when compared with past approaches based on public campaigns is set out in Fig. 4.8.

Social marketing has three characteristics: it aims to achieve a particular 'social good' (rather than commercial benefit) with specific behavioural goals clearly identified and targeted; it is a systematic process phased to address short-, medium- and long-term issues; and it utilizes a range of marketing techniques and approaches (a 'marketing mix').

Here the 'social good' can be articulated in terms of achieving specific, achievable and measurable behavioural goals, relevant to improving heath and well-being[52].

If you want to read more about social marketing, there is a useful pocket guide[53] available on http://www.nsms.org.uk

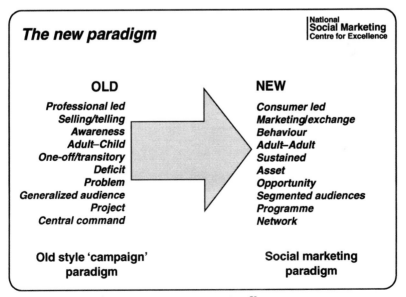

Fig. 4.8 Social marketing compared with campaigns[53].

Undertaking clinical audit and health equity audit

Clinical audit

The clinical audit cycle (Fig. 4.9) refers to the monitoring of performance against pre-defined standards. Measurement of one's performance against defined criteria can be demanding, but the real challenge is to make necessary adjustments and re-evaluate your performance—in other words to complete the cycle (see Box 4.19).

Standards are developed for the NHS through NSFs. NICE evaluates new technologies and develops guidelines. Progress on the implementation of clinical governance is monitored at all levels of the health service by the Health Care Commission. The involvement of patients and public is promoted at both a local and national level. Annual surveys of users form part of the monitoring process.

The National Patient Safety Agency (NPSA) is a Special Health Authority which was created to coordinate the efforts of all those involved in health care, and more importantly to learn from patient safety incidents occurring in the NHS. As well as making sure that incidents are reported in the first place, the NPSA promotes an open culture across the health service, encouraging doctors and other staff to report incidents and 'near misses', when things almost go wrong. A key aim is to encourage staff to report incidents without fear of personal reprimand and know that by sharing their experiences others will be able to learn lessons and improve patient safety. The NPSA also supports local organizations in addressing their concerns about the performance of individual doctors and dentists, through its responsibility for the National Clinical Assessment Service (NCAS), formerly known as the National Clinical Assessment Authority.

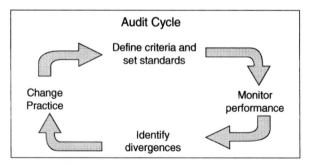

Fig. 4.9 The clinical audit cycle.

Box 4.19 A routine example of clinical audit from frontline general practice

One criterion used to assess the quality of care provided for people with hypertension is the proportion of patients whose blood pressures lie below 150/90 mmHg (140/85 for people with diabetes). Under their new contract, general practice teams are rewarded for achieving a target of 70 per cent of people with hypertension thus controlled (the standard). In this instance, the practice was surprised to find that they were only achieving 64 per cent coverage. On closer examination of data, it transpired that coverage among hypertensive patients attending the branch surgery sited on a deprived estate was only 45 per cent. Furthermore, only 3 per cent of the patients of Doctor X who works predominantly from this site were adequately controlled.

Various interventions were made to tackle these divergences. The clinical audit lead decided to monitor performance more closely. Patients whose blood pressure remained elevated and who had not been seen in the last 6 months were contacted by letter and asked to attend surgery. Doctor X was provided with a copy of the practice hypertension protocol (based on the British Society of Hypertension's guidelines) and asked to dedicate more time to this area of his clinical practice. The records of patients in the target group were tagged electronically so as to ease their identification at opportunistic consultation. More nurse time was channelled to supporting the branch surgery.

Regular monthly monitoring and sharing of the results across the team over the next half year revealed gratifying improvements. Six months later, coverage rates among Doctor X's patients and the branch surgery were 62 and 66 per cent, respectively; across the practice as a whole the 70 per cent target was achieved.

Following Dr Harold Shipman's murder of at least 215 of his own patients, the Baker report recommended routine monitoring of general practice mortality rates[54]. Despite some encouraging pilot studies, no practical method of mortality monitoring has yet been agreed. Unusual mortality rates are mostly the result of unmeasured case mix factors (demography and deprivation) affecting practices[55]. The Shipman Inquiry[56] has made extensive recommendations regarding the future workings of the General Medical Council and, specifically, has sought more stringent processes of medical revalidation.

Doing a health equity audit

As with clinical audit, the intention of health equity audit is not only to measure baseline differences between different population groups but also to act before measuring again, i.e. to complete the cycle. Like clinical audit, it is therefore a tool for making change happen. The technique has been developed to identify how fairly services or other resources are distributed in relation to the health needs of different population groups or geographical areas. The purpose of a health equity audit is to help services narrow health inequalities by using evidence on inequalities to inform decisions on investment, service planning, commissioning and delivery, and to review the impact of action on inequalities[57]. In England, equity audit is mandatory for PCTs.

Examples of ways a primary health care team might address inequities in access to their services include:

+ Ethnic monitoring in large, heterogeneous practice populations to answer questions such as whether the patients on our diabetes register are representative of the practice population. Alternatively, are we failing to detect early cases in, for example, South Asian groups?

+ Identifying a service lead for people with learning difficulties, a priority group that has repeatedly been found to receive substandard primary care

+ Coordinated case management with local community mental health teams for care of the severely mentally ill

+ The 'basics'—appropriate use of interpreters, signage, translated leaflets— for patients who do not speak English.

We give an example of a health equity audit of heart failure management in general practice in Chapter 6.

Evaluating

How do we know whether our interventions are having the desired effect? Clinicians can monitor the impact of treatments on an individual patient basis, but how do we examine the impact of a new service or screening programme? In this section, we will look first at what is meant by quality of care and consider one well-known framework for its evaluation. We then consider how quality of care is promoted across the NHS as a whole.

Quality of care and its evaluation

Quality in health care means doing the right thing, at the right time, in the right way, to the right person—and having the best possible result. A more formal framework is provided by Maxwell[58] who described six dimensions to quality:

- Effectiveness (achieves intended benefit)
- Acceptability (satisfies reasonable expectations)
- Efficiency (resources not oversupplied to some patients to the detriment of others)
- Accessibility (those who need services will receive them)
- Equity (resources are fairly shared)
- Relevance (treatments are appropriate to their particular target groups).

Of course, it is not only health professionals who are interested in the quality of care they provide—as media interest in medical mishaps reminds us. Managers in hospitals and health authorities are charged to monitor quality as part of clinical governance (see below). Whether as users or voters, the general population have great interest in quality of health care and may have different priorities from those of doctors. As we described in Chapter 3, they may place clear information, caring communication and outcomes that improve activities of daily living higher up their list than technical aspects of care which may be difficult for them to assess.

Evaluation has been defined as 'a process that attempts to determine as systematically and objectively as possible the relevance, effectiveness and impact of activities in the light of their objectives, e.g. evaluation of structure, process and outcome, clinical trials, quality of care'. Where do we start when thinking about evaluation of a delivery system in the NHS? Avedis Donabedian distinguished four elements[59]:

- Structure (buildings, staff, equipment)
- Process (all that is done to patients)
- Outputs (immediate results of medical intervention)
- Outcomes (gains in health status).

Thus, for example, early evaluation of the new national screening programme for colonic cancer may consider

- The volume and costs of new equipment (colonoscopic, radiographic, histopathological), staff and buildings (structure)
- The numbers of patients screened, coverage rates within a defined age range, numbers of true- and false-positives (process)
- Number of cancers identified, operations performed (outputs)
- Complication rates, colonic cancer incidence, prevalence and mortality rates (outcomes).

This distinction is helpful because for many interventions it may be difficult to obtain robust data on health outcomes unless large numbers are scrutinized over long periods. For example, evaluating the quality of hypertension management within a general practice, you may be reliant on intermediate outcome or process measures (the proportion of the appropriate population screened, treated and adequately controlled) as a proxy for the health status outcomes. The assumption here is that evidence from larger scale studies showing that control of hypertension reduces subsequent death rates from heart disease will be reflected in your own practice populations' health experience.

Thinking about the care provided for people with a particular disease, evaluation can be considered in terms of different elements of their care: prevention, diagnosis, treatment and rehabilitation. Table 4.9 gives examples of measures the effectiveness of specific interventions.

Table 4.9 Examples of measures that might be relevant for evaluation

Smoking cessation service	Number of smokers seen and counselled
	Prescriptions for nicotine replacement therapy dispensed
	Quit rates, costs (of material/staff, etc.)
	Trends in smoking prevalence
	Death rates from smoking-related diseases.
Immunization programmes	Numbers of vaccines administered
	Proportion of target population covered
	Costs (of vaccines distributed, maintaining cold chain other disposables, staff deployed, etc.)
	Disease incidence rates over time.
Breast screening programme	Numbers of mammograms carried out
	Abnormality detection rates
	False positives at lumpectomy
	Proportion of target population covered, breast cancer incidence (falling or rising?)
	Long term-mortality trends
	Costs
Cardiac rehabilitation services	Numbers passing through programme
	Numbers as a proportion of all patients admitted with diagnosis of myocardial infarction, and as a proportion of all of those meeting appropriate referral criteria
	Percentages of patients in programme receiving recommended interventions post-myocardial infarction (aspirin, beta-blockers, statins if not contraindicated)
	Impact on patients' quality of life
	Costs
	Long term re-infarction rates
	Mortality rates post-myocardial infarction

Table 4.9 *(continued)* Examples of measures that might be relevant for evaluation

Hip replacement for osteoarthritis	Numbers of operations performed
	Lengths of stay
	Infection or other complication rates
	Readmission rates
	Proportion of patients requiring surgical revision
	Costs (prostheses, hospital stay and rehab)
	Numbers on waiting lists
	Length of waiting
	Prevalence of unmet need within local community
	Patient satisfaction surveys
	Impact on quality of life/activities of daily living
Chronic disease management (e.g. diabetes at general practice level)	Numbers on disease register
	Proportion receiving annual check (e.g. retinal screening)
	Proportion meeting appropriate standards for criteria of good care (e.g. blood pressure below 140/90 mmHg, Hba1c <7, etc.)
	Proportion of patients with management plan
	Costs
	Rates of disease-related complications

One of the biggest problems in evaluating large-scale public health interventions is the confounding effect of the many different factors influencing outcomes: background 'noise'. For example, assessing the impact of mass media campaigns against smoking might be complicated by the impact of new laws to prevent smoking in public places, changes to the national curriculum, increased taxation on cigarettes or background declines in the population prevalence of smoking. Measures of outcome may be limited. Readily available measures of quality are not necessarily the most important, and the most important elements of quality may not be easily measurable. It is important not to fall into the trap of going for the easily measured as this will result in the programme focusing on achieving that particular measure at the expense of the more important ones. The long time lag between intervention and effect also poses difficulty. With their interest in equity of provision, public health specialists have to consider the accessibility of services particularly to disadvantaged groups.

Clinical governance

A common criticism of much of what doctors do to try and improve the quality of their care is that it is piecemeal and poorly coordinated. Variable quality of care, particularly in the poorest, least healthy and least well resourced parts of the country, has long been a fact of NHS life (an example of Julian Tudor Hart's 'inverse care law'). *A First Class Service*[60], published by the Labour government in 1998, contained a blueprint for improving quality encapsulated in Fig. 4.10.

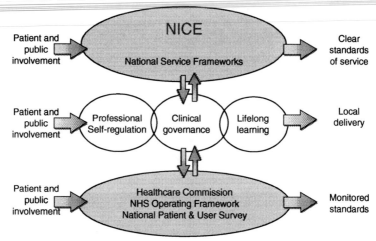

Fig. 4.10 Standards for the NHS[60].

The term 'clinical governance' (borrowing on notions of corporate governance from the private sector) was coined to refer to the framework through which NHS organizations and their staff are accountable for the quality of patient care. It covers the organizations, systems and processes for monitoring and improving services. The different components of clinical governance are listed below:

Processes for quality improvement

1. Patient and public involvement
2. Risk management
3. Clinical audit
4. Clinical effectiveness programmes
5. Staffing and staff management

Staff focus

6. Education, training and continuing personal and professional development

Information

7. Use of information to support clinical governance and health care delivery

Standards are developed for the NHS through NSFs and other national policy documents. The NICE evaluates new technologies and develops guidelines. Progress on the implementation of clinical governance is monitored at all levels of the health service by the Health Care Commission. The involvement of patients and public is promoted both at a local and a national level. Annual surveys of users form part of the monitoring process.

Further resources

Oxford Handbook of Public Health Practice[61]
Oxford Handbook of General Practice[62]
Modernisation Agency. *Improvement Leaders' Guides*[63]
NHS Modernisation Agency. *Improvement Leaders' Guide. Involving Patients and Carers*[26]
Managing Change in the NHS[64]
Prime Minister's Strategy Unit. *Strategy Survival Guide*[38]
The Improvement Leaders' Guide Managing the Human Dimension of Change[65]
Leadership in public health practice[16]
Neil Goodwin. Leadership in public health. In: Griffiths S, Hunter D, ed. *New Perspectives in Public Health*[20].

References

1. Heller T, Hill A, Lloyd C, Allen A. *Public Health. Towards a Social Model of Health Policy and Provision*. Milton Keynes: The Open University, 2001; 99–137.
2. Gray JAM. A National Public Health Knowledge Service. *ph.com* 6[4], 4. 2005. London: Faculty of Public Health.
3. Bingham P. *An Introduction to Quality and Outcome Framework Data. 7*. INphoRM. Cambridge: Eastern Region Public Health Observatory, 2006.
4. Bower P, Mead N, Roland M. What dimensions underlie patients' responses to the general practice assessment survey? A factor analytic study. *Family Practice* 2002; 19: 489–495.
5. Safran GD, Kosinski M, Tarlov AR, Rogers WH, Taira DA, Lieberman N, *et al*. The primary care assessment study. Tests of data quality and measurement performance. *Medical Care* 1998; 36: 728–729.
6. Chanter C, Ashmore S, Mandair S. Improving the patient experience in general practice with the general practice assessment questionnaire (GPAQ). *Quality and Primary Care* 2005; 13: 225–232.
7. Begg NT, Gill ON, White JM. COVER (Cover of Vaccination Evaluated Rapidly): Description of the England and Wales scheme. *Public Health* 1989; 103: 81–89.
8. Deckers JG, Paget WJ, Schellevis FG, Fleming DM. European primary care surveillance networks: their structure and operation. *Family Practice* 2006; 23: 151–158.
9. Doroshenko A, Cooper D, Smith GE, Gerrard E, Verlander FQ, Nicoll A. Evaluation of syndromic surveillance based on National Health Service Direct data—England and Wales. *MMWR* 2005; 54: 161–166.
10. Brice A, Burls A, Hill A. Finding and appraising evidence. In: Pencheon D, Melzer D, Gray M, Guest C, ed. *Oxford Handbook of Public Health Practice*, 2nd edn. Oxford: Oxford University Press, 2006; 184–192.
11. Greenhalgh T, Hurwitz B. *Narrative Based Medicine: Dialogue and Discourse in Clinical Practice*. London: BMA Books, 1998.
12. Oxman AD, Sackett DL, Guyatt GH. The Evidence-Based Medicine Working Group. Users' guides to the medical literature. I. How to get started. *Journal of the American Medical Association* 1993; 270: 2093–2095.

13. Gray JAM. *Evidence-based Healthcare*, 2nd edn. London; Churchill Livingstone, 2001.

14. Straus SE, Richardson WS, Glasziou P, Haynes RB. *Evidence Based Medicine*, 3rd edn. London: Churchill Livingstone, 2005.

15. Greenhalgh T. *How to Read a Paper: The Basics of Evidence Based Medicine*, 2nd edn. London: BMJ Books; 2000.

16. Pointer D, Sanchez JP. Leadership in public health practice. In: Scutchfield FD, Keck CW, ed. *Principles of Public Health Practice*. New York: Thomson Delmar Learning, 2003; 140–159.

17. Bennis W, Nanus B. Leaders. New York: Harper Collins; 1996.

18. Crainer S, Dearlove D. *The Future of Leadership*. London, NHS Institute for Innovation and Improvement, 2005.

19. Klein KJ, Ziegert JC, Knight AP, Xiao Y. Dynamic delegation: shared, hierarchical, and deindividualised leadership in extreme action teams. *Administrative Science Quarterly* 2006; in press.

20. Goodwin N. Leadership in public health. In: Griffiths S, Hunter D, ed. *New Perspectives in Public Health*. 2nd edn. Oxford: Radcliffe Publishing, 2006; 330–337.

21. Hunter DJ. Management and public health. In: Detels R, McEwen J, Beaglehole R, Tanaka H, ed. *Oxford Textbook of Public Health*, 4th edn. Oxford: Oxford University Press, 2002; 921–935.

22. Thorpe A. Networks. In: Griffiths S, Hunter D, ed. *New Perspectives in Public Health*. Oxford: Radcliffe Publishing, 2006; 338–347.

23. Hunter DJ. *Public Health Policy*. Cambridge: Polity Press, 2003.

24. Coulter A. *Engaging Patients in their Healthcare. How is the UK Doing Relative to Other Countries?* Oxford: Picker Institute Europe, 2006.

25. Department of Health. *A Stronger Local Voice: A Framework for Creating a Stronger Local Voice in the Development of Health and Social Care Services*. London: Department of Health, 2006.

26. NHS Modernisation Agency. *Improvement Leaders' Guide. Involving Patients and Carers*. London: Department of Health, 2005.

27. Greco M, Carter M. *Improving Practice Questionnaire (IPQ) Tool Kit*. Chichester, UK: Aeneas Press, 2002.

28. Picker Institute Europe. *Picker General Practice Questionnaire*. Oxford, Picker Institute Europe, 2004.

29. Murray SA, Tapson J, McCullum J, Little A, Department of Health. Listening to local voices: adapting rapid appraisal to assess health and social needs in general practice. The new NHS modern dependable. *British Medical Journal* 1994; 308: 698–700.

30. Ham C. Tragic choices in healthcare: lessons from the Child B case. *British Medical Journal* 1999; 319: 1258–1261.

31. Griffiths S, Jewell T, Hope T. Setting priorities in health care. In: Pencheon D, Melzer D, Gray M, Guest C, ed. *Oxford Handbook of Public Health Practice*, 2nd edn. Oxford: Oxford University Press, 2006; 404–410.

32. Wright J, Kyle D. Assessing health needs. In: Pencheon D, Melzer D, Gray M, Guest C, ed. *Oxford Handbook of Public Health Practice*, 2nd edn. Oxford: Oxford University Press, 2006; 29–31.

33. Wright J, Williams R, Wilkinson JR. Health needs assessment: development and importance of health needs assessment. *British Medical Journal* 1998; 316: 1310–1313.

34. Health Development Agency. *Introducing Health Impact Assessment (HIA): Informing the Decision-making Process.* Taylor L, Blair-Stevens C, ed. London, Health Development Agency, 2002.

35. Scott-Samuel A, Arden K. Assessing health impacts on a population. In: Pencheon D, Melzer D, Gray M, Guest C, editors. *Oxford Handbook of Public Health Practice,* 2nd edn. Oxford: Oxford University Press, 2006; 42–55.

36. Rogers E. *The Diffusion of Innovation.* 4th edn. New York: Free Press, 1995.

37. Gladwell M. *The Tipping Point. How Little Things Can Make a Big Difference.* London: Abacus, 2000.

38. Prime Minister's Strategy Unit. *Strategy Survival Guide Version 2.1.* 2004.

39. Freeman R, Gillam S, Epstein L, Plamping D. *Community Oriented Primary Care. A Resource for Developers.* London: King's Fund, 1994.

40. Prochaska J, DiClemente C. Stages and processes of self-change of smoking: towards an integrated model of change. *Journal of Consulting and Clinical Psychology* 1983; 51: 390–395.

41. Rollnick S, Mason P, Butler C. *Health Behaviour Change. A Guide for Practitioners.* Edinburgh: Churchill Livingstone; 2005.

42. Edwards A, Hood K, Matthews E, Russell D, Russell I, Barker J, *et al.* The effectiveness of one-to-one risk communication interventions in health care: a systematic review. *Medical Decision Making* 2000; 20: 290–297.

43. Budescu DV, Weinberg S, Allsten TS. Decisions based on numerically and verbally expressed uncertainties. *Journal of Experimental Psychology-General* 1988; 14: 281–294.

44. Wilson DK, Purdon SE, Wallston KA. Compliance to health recommendations: a theoretical overview of message framing. *Health Education Testing* 1988; 3: 161–171.

45. Slater E. How risks of breast cancer and benefits of screening are communicated to women: analysis of 58 pamphlets. *British Medical Journal* 1998; 317: 263–264.

46. Fahey T, Griffiths S, Peters TJ. Evidence based purchasing: understanding results of clinical trials and systematic reviews. *British Medical Journal* 1995; 311: 1056–1059.

47. Edwards A, Elwyn G, Mulley A. Explaining risks: turning numerical data into meaningful pictures. *British Medical Journal* 2002; 324: 827–830.

48. Lipkus IM, Hollands JG. The visual communication of risk. *Journal of the National Cancer Institute Monographs* 1999; 25: 149–163.

49. Harrabin R, Coote A, Allen J. *Health in the News: Risk, Reporting and Media Influence.* London: King's Fund, 2003.

50. Department of Health. *Delivering Choosing Health: Making Healthier Choices Easier.* London, Department of Health, 2005.

51. Deparment of Health. *Our Health, Our Care, Our Say: A New Direction for Community Services.* Cm 6737 ed. London: Department of Health, 2006.

52. Department of Health, National Consumer Council. *Realising the Potential of Effective Social Marketing.* London: Department of Health; 2005.

53. National Social Marketing Centre for Excellence. *Social Marketing. Pocket Guide.* London: Department of Health, 2005.

54. Baker R. *Harold Shipman's Clinical Practice 1974–1998: A Clinical Audit Commissioned by the Chief Medical Officer.* Norwich: Stationery Office, 2001.

55. Mohammed M, Booth K, Marshall D, Brolly M, Marshall T, Cheng KK, *et al.* A practical method for monitoring general practice mortality in the UK: findings from a pilot

study in a health board of Northern Ireland. *British Journal of General Practice* 2005; 518: 670–676.

56. **The Shipman Inquiry.** *Safeguarding Patients: Lessons from the Past, Proposals for the Future.* London: The Stationery Office, 2004.

57. **Department of Health.** *Health Equity Audit: A Guide for the NHS.* London: Department of Health, 2003.

58. **Maxwell R.** Quality assessment in health. *British Medical Journal* 1984; 288: 1470–1472.

59. **Donabedian A.** *The Definition of Quality and Approaches to its Assessment.* Ann Arbor, MI: Health Administration Press, 1980.

60. **Department of Health.** *A First Class Service: Quality in the New NHS.* London: Department of Health, 1998.

61. **Pencheon D, Melzer D, Gray M, Guest C.** *Oxford Handbook of Public Health Practice,* 2nd edn. Oxford: Oxford University Press, 2006.

62. **Simon C, Everitt H, Kendrick T.** *Oxford Handbook of General Practice,* 2nd edn. Oxford: Oxford University Press, 2005.

63. **Modernisation Agency.** *Improvement Leaders' Guides.* Modernisation Agency, 2002.

64. **Iles V, Sutherland K.** *Managing Change in the NHS: Organisational Change.* London: National Co-ordinating Centre for NHS Service Delivery and Organisation, 2001.

65. **NHS Modernisation Agency.** *Improvement Leaders' Guides. Managing the Human Dimensions of Change.* NHS Modernisation Agency, 2005.

5

Public health in practice: improving health

This chapter has been written with input from Tony Jewell, Chief Medical Officer, Welsh Assembly Government, and former GP

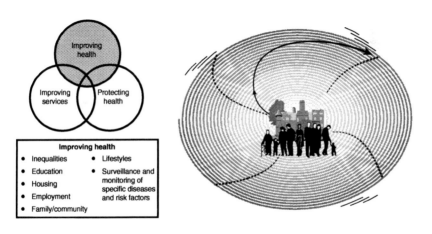

This chapter addresses the first of the three domains of public health practice, improving health, and is concerned with the broader influences on health.

In this chapter we use case studies to demonstrate that good health is achieved by the efforts of many, amongst whom primary care health services play a key role not only in providing good quality clinical care but also through providing support to the wider community. This underlines the relevance of the population based approach to primary care. Improving health is part and parcel of everyday care and integral to providing the package of services within the community, taking account not only of prevention but of care and support.

Health improvement is concerned with promoting healthier lifestyles both through addressing the wider determinants of health and through promoting individual behaviour change. It requires close working between primary care teams and public health specialists, and between primary care organizations (PCOs) and partners such as local authorities and the voluntary sector (see Chapters 3 and 4). For example, reducing obesity in a local population will involve Directors of Public Health (DsPH) and their teams in leading local strategies, but will also involve schools and teachers in providing healthy school food and education as well as encouraging school sports and promoting healthier lifestyles. School nurses and health visitors will work with children and their families to provide health checks and advice, and engage local shops in playing a role by providing healthy choices. Clinicians have a role to play both through giving advice to their patients on losing weight and the obesity-related risks of heart disease and, where necessary, prescribing or providing clinical interventions.

Earlier chapters have described the policy and strategy backgrounds of the key elements of health improvement as:

- Supporting a positive, holistic approach to health
- Addressing health inequalities through positive actions to break the cycle of deprivation
- Addressing the health impact of determinants such as housing and employment to create healthy sustainable environments
- Utilizing education and modern approaches to communication, such as social marketing, to promote health at both individual and societal level
- Promoting healthy lifestyles through individually focused health education and lifestyle advice
- Building healthy communities and developing social capital.

In practice, this means that the local primary care provider organization (the GP practice) becomes the population of interest, concerned not only with those who access services but also those who do not, e.g. those who benefit from prevention initiatives. Health visitors and other practice-based staff will be concerned not only with what goes on in the GP surgery but with the community services available to their populations such as playgroups, community projects, employment advice and young people's services, looking beyond the individual doctor: patient consultation. Tudor Hart in *A New Kind of Doctor* was one of the first to pioneer this concept[1].

Examples of how this can be translated into practice at a local level for GPs and their practices is illustrated in Table 5.1.

Table 5.1 Characteristics of health improvement at a local level

Characteristic of health improvement	Example from primary care
Supporting a positive holistic approach to health	Taking a whole person perspective in providing lifestyle advice. For example, giving advice about benefits and finance or how to access further educational opportunities when attending surgery.
Addressing health inequalities through positive actions to break the cycle of deprivation	Providing help to young teenage mothers and their babies through a support group which meets regularly at the health centre; signposting them to other agencies and services if needed.
Utilizing education and modern approaches to communication to promote health both at individual and societal level	Linking between the primary care team and local schools to provide support for health promotion in the school. Having available computer programs tailored to the interests of young men, e.g. using sports images and messages, highlighting the risks of unsafe sex and abuse of alcohol. Finding ways of using social marketing techniques in a local campaign to promote uptake of services such as antenatal care, smoking cessation and immunization. Regular meetings between school nurse and school governors about healthy school policies.
Addressing the health impact of determinants such as housing; and employment to create healthy sustainable environments	Making sure housing advice is available in the practice as well as the surgery, signposting to local authority housing benefits, or citizens advice bureaux for debt counselling.
Promoting healthy lifestyles through individually focused health education and lifestyle advice	Give advice during routine consultations about integrating physical activity into daily living. Referral for exercise to local leisure centre; providing smoking cessation advice.
Building healthy communities and developing social capital	Getting to know local councillors, engaging in public consultation, being part of voluntary activities in the community and supporting local community groups.

The approaches of health improvement are fundamental to public health and reflect international initiatives spelt out, for example, in the Ottawa and Bangkok Charters (see Chapter 1).

Improving health is not a set of either/or choices. Approaches need to combine advice to individuals whilst at the same time creating circumstances which are conducive to better health within communities. As described in Chapter 1, improved health results from interactions at individual, local, national and global levels (see Fig. 5.1).

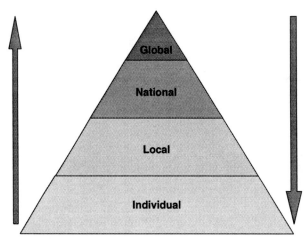

Fig. 5.1 Multilevel approach in a global context.

Prevention is at the heart of health improvement. In Chapter 1, we describe the three levels of prevention, and in Chapter 7 make the case for prevention as a key part of clinical practice. The Wanless Report[2], which we discussed in Chapter 1, emphasized that prevention needs to be at the forefront not only of the work of public health practitioners but of all health care workers, particularly those in primary care.

This is reinforced in the most recent English White Paper 'Our Health, Our Care, Our Say'[3]. In its summary, it boldly states that:

> Health and social care services will provide better prevention services with earlier intervention. GP practices and Primary Care Trusts (PCTs) will work much more closely with local government services to ensure that there is early support for prevention.

The following statements commit the government to doing more to tackle inequalities/disparities in health and health care and to improving access to community services.

> We will ensure that local health and social care commissioners work together to understand and address local inequalities. ... We will increase the quantity and quality of primary care in under-served, deprived areas. And we will ensure that people with particular needs get the services they require – young people, mothers, ethnic

minorities, people with disabilities, people at the end of their lives, offenders and others. To do this, it will be necessary to reorientate our health and social care services to focus together on prevention and health promotion.

These words, if turned into action, will influence both attitudes towards and delivery of health services. They will raise the profile of prevention in primary and secondary care, as well as promoting ongoing community-based care. However, good words are fine but there will always be the risk that the pressures of the acute services once more dominate the agenda; government support will be needed to develop community-based approaches which underpin health-improving strategies. This will in turn need to be supported by redirection of resources and by strengthening capacity within local communities. As such, this is not a new challenge nor a new direction. It represents a reinforcement of community development approaches and their important role in creating and promoting health.

Community development has been defined as 'building active and sustainable communities based on social justice and mutual respect. ... changing power structures to remove the barriers that prevent people from participating in the issues which affect their lives'[4].

Healthy Living Centres (HLCs) are a good example of the community development approach. They were funded from the lottery between 2002 and 2005 and administered by the New Opportunities Fund, now the Big Lottery (www. biglotteryfund.org.uk). HLCs were established in deprived areas across the UK. The specifications for the projects reflected the needs of the different local communities. The programme covered a wide range of initiatives from educational theatre for schools to walks for the elderly and community cafes serving healthy food. Many HLCs were closely linked to local primary care services, providing outreach smoking cessation, exercise classes for older people and in some instances the opportunity to rebuild primary care facilities at the heart of communities (see the case study on Bromley by Bow healthy living centre in Chapter 3).

The HLC programme has been evaluated by a network of researchers, the Bridge Consortium. Their second annual report (available on the Big Lottery website) describes the many achievements of the programme including the breadth of activities, wide engagement of local people and effective targeting of parts of the community not usually reached[5]. However, the report also highlights the problems, many of which local PCTs will be only too aware of, of bridging cultures and of the difficulties sustaining momentum particularly when faced with local structural/managerial changes and of securing long-term funding.

Along with other neighbourhood initiatives, HLCs contribute to a sense of networking and belonging sometimes called social capital. The notion of social capital is useful as a way of describing the advantages to be gained for local populations by developing and supporting local activities which engage a range of partners. The concept refers 'to features of social organisations, such as trust, norms and networks that can improve the efficiency of society by facilitating coordinated actions'[6]. Social capital may be associated with better health because it enables disadvantaged groups to access material resources through connections to socially advantaged groups. It is also relevant to the principle of civil society—meaning collective or group action around shared interests, purposes and values by a diverse grouping which can include voluntary organizations, faith communities, local businesses, trade unions, professional groups and others committed to sharing actions which will promote good health in the community.

These concepts of community development, social capital and civil society translate into every day practice for primary care as:

+ A clear focus on reducing heath inequalities and social disparities

+ New ways of working within practices and a greater focus on prevention

+ Closer working with local communities

+ Closer working between DsPH and local practices, often joint appointments

+ Closer working with local authorities on Local Strategic Partnerships, Local Area Agreements and other joint initiatives

+ New ways of working with other health care partners through commissioning to monitor outcomes (practice-based commissioning oriented towards prevention and health improvement)

+ Reorientation of training to ensure appropriate skills amongst all staff.

What does this mean in practice?

We will illustrate key approaches to health improvement through a series of local case studies.

Case study 1: teenage pregnancy

One of the major challenges for the UK is its very high rate of teenage pregnancy and the associated cycle of deprivation. Not only are young teen mothers at risk, but so are their children who tend to have higher rates of infection, sudden infant death and recurrent hospital admission[7].

Box 5.1 Maggie

Maggie is 16. She has a 1-year-old son Darren. Maggie got pregnant accidently, having unprotected sex after an evening binge drinking with mates at the local club. She did not tell her mum until it was too late for an abortion and, anyway, she quite wanted the baby although her boyfriend Tom disappeared off the scene pretty quickly once she told him she was pregnant. Maggie skipped school once she knew she was having a baby and never went back. She fell out with her mum so she is living in a damp bedsit with Darren and living off benefits. She is waiting for the council to find her a flat. Meanwhile, she shares a kitchen with others in the house. She eats lots of fast food because it is easier than cooking—and she is smoking heavily. She feels pretty low a lot of the time and does not really know where life is taking her. Darren has been in hospital several times with gastroenteritis and also chest problems.

There are many young teenagers like Maggie who are in need of help and ongoing support from primary care not just with the physical and emotional problems they and their babies face but with their social needs—education, housing, financial and social support. Groups who are more vulnerable to becoming teenage parents include those who are: in or leaving care; underachieving at school; involved in crime; living in areas of higher deprivation; homeless; and members of some ethnic groups[8]. The evidence shows that teen mothers are more likely to:

- Book later in pregnancy for antenatal care to the health service, missing out on preventive interventions such as folic acid supplements
- To smoke
- Have stressful relationships during pregnancy
- Move house during pregnancy
- Have low incomes (90 per cent on income support)
- Give birth to low birth weight babies who also have a higher infant mortality rate
- Have a higher child mortality (1–3 years) among their children
- Have their children admitted to hospital with accidents and gastroenteritis
- Not breast feed.

The UK has one of the highest teenage birth and abortion rates in Western Europe[9]. This vulnerable group of young women, their partners and their children have been the focus of public health programmes, for example Sure Start (www.surestart.gov.uk), which have the specific objective of breaking the cycle of deprivation by positive intervention. However, primary care interventions start with primary prevention, including health education and provision of appropriate and accessible contraception services. These may be in GPs surgeries but also across other settings including schools, youth clubs and young people's family planning services.

In cases where young women wish to continue their pregnancy, special attention needs to be provided to meet their needs and ensure maximum support during pregnancy and in preparation for child care. An attached midwife may need to monitor carefully attendance at antenatal clinics and provide advice not only on the physical aspects but also on day to day issues.

Some ways in which the contributions of a population-based perspective can support the primary care team in meeting the needs of an individual teen mother are summarized in Table 5.2.

Table 5.2 Roles of public health and primary care in supporting teenage mothers

Concerns	Population issues/public health programmes	Individual issues/primary care interventions
Maggie		
Teen mother without social support	Assess needs of teen mothers in local community; define any gaps, e.g. in in service provision for contraception, emergency contraception	Provide antenatal care Parenting classes in the practice
	Ensure good antenatal and postnatal care through commissioning contracts	Support during delivery Antenatal and postnatal support from attached midwife/health visitor/GP
Education	Work with education authorities on health and lifestyle education in schools as a preventive strategy	Make close links with local schools
	Work with education authorities on opportunities for further education plus childcare to allow return to education	Provide information on educational opportunities
Damp housing	Work with local government/ housing NGOs to provide good quality housing	Referral to housing department

Table 5.2 *(continued)* Roles of public health and primary care in supporting teenage mothers

Concerns	Population issues/public health programmes	Individual issues/primary care interventions
Poor diet	Promote healthy eating through local/national campaigns. Identify whether easier access to healthier food can be promoted	Advice from health visitor/ community worker/ dietician
Lack of exercise	Promote health benefits of physical activity through media/local campaigns; work with local planners on safe play areas	Advice from health visitor/ others in primary care team including social worker
Smoking	Ensure smoking cessation services are accessible and appropriate; evaluate impact and continuously improve quality	Refer to smoking cessation support services; reinforce with advice from all health care professionals
Alcohol	Put in place community-wide strategies to educate about sensible drinking.	Provide advice and counselling about safe drinking especially risks of alcohol during pregnancy
	Consider policies to protect young people from alcohol-related harm, e.g. Saturday night city centre initiatives	Access to post coital contraception
No money	Support development of parent-friendly employment	Give information about available benefits; job-seeking opportunities and childcare. Links to social worker who can provide support
Depressed	Develop strategy for detection and support of mothers with postnatal depression, arguing for resources based on evidence of effective interventions	Provide support and treatment if necessary; arrange for social support through Sure Start/ local mother and toddler group
Darren		
Frequent hospital admissions with infections	Local environmental health officers can help maintain standards in multiple occupancy housing where teen mothers may be placed	Promote breast feeding Advice on hygiene, cooking, etc. Case conference between paediatricians and primary care team if admissions are repeated
No play space and lack of stimulation	Local authority planners create safe play spaces for children	Refer to Sure Start or local mother and toddler group
Risk of non-accidental injury (NAI)	Surveillance of NAI	Assess to see if should be on at-risk register

Case study 2: homelessness

The problems of homelessness and rough sleeping provide another set of issues which require complementary population and primary care perspectives. Although the numbers sleeping rough have reduced thanks to the government's active approach to reducing rough sleeping, there are many young men who have some or all of the features of a chaotic lifestyle highlighted by Gary's story and who may well be homeless and without social support, sleeping rough from time to time. The complex inter-relationships between mental health, personal security, abuse of alcohol and drugs can only be addressed by working with different groups in different sectors who have the skills needed for each individual in need of care.

Box 5.2 Gary

Gary is 25 years old and is currently unemployed and homeless. He is on probation following arrest for shoplifting. He has a drugs habit and is also clinically depressed and feels he is useless. He grew up in a violent household, often witnessing his dad hitting his mum, and spent some time in care. His mother has now left his father to go back home abroad. He left school with one GCSE and has never had a job. Last year he was in prison, not for the first time, for shoplifting—a short sentence which meant he lost his flat when his girlfriend moved away. One of the good things about being in prison was he was able to see a dentist, but he is now confused about how to get more care. He sleeps rough when he does not have the money to get into the night shelter and finds it difficult to keep the appointments made for him with his care worker.

We know from the literature that certain groups are most at risk of becoming homeless, particularly young people who have been in care. They are particularly vulnerable around the time they begin to live independently. Other groups at risk of homelessness include those with mental illnesses and those with substance abuse problems. Problems of homelessness also affect migrant and refugee groups as well as ex-servicemen.

Table 5.3 describes contributions from population and individual perspectives.

The list of issues and actions is not exhaustive but from both public health and primary care perspectives it is important that there is a well coordinated response to Gary's needs. There is always a risk of too many agencies being involved and too many people addressing their specific issues without considering the total package of support needed by Gary and the usefulness of a key worker through whom others need to work. Patients such as Gary highlight the need for primary health care workers to know not only about clinical issues or local hospital services but also local voluntary groups and services who provide essential help and support. In areas where there are groups of recidivist homeless, often with alcohol- and drug-related problems, special services may be the best model of care to provide[10].

Close links between practices and mental health teams as well as with A&E departments can help to ensure appropriate referrals and care plans. Links between health and the criminal justice system are important, for example between the local prison and the PCT or between the practice team and the local probation service, and good communication with the local police can make it easier to handle cases of domestic violence more sensitively.

Table 5.3 Roles of public health and primary care in supporting the homeless

Concerns	Population issues/public health programmes	Individual issues/primary care interventions
Gary		
Drugs problem	Ensure school-based programmes of health education also reach children in care	Identify key worker and mobilize primary care team, members with appropriate expertise
	Organize needle exchange schemes; consider PMS scheme with local practices	Education re risks of HIV/AIDS Provide support to come off drugs
	Work with NGOs on strategic approach Support development of local initiatives involving Drugs Action Team with partners, monitor their impact, participate in commissioning plans to bridge between health and social care Ensure protocols for referrals to all partners: hospital trusts, social services, drug and alcohol services, voluntary sector, faith communities	Identify key players in local voluntary groups who can work with practice staff
Depression	Plan appropriate services within primary care and also with specialist support	Work with mental health team to provide appropriate support and counselling

(Continued)

Table 5.3 (continued) Roles of public health and primary care in supporting the homeless

Concerns	Population issues/public health programmes	Individual issues/primary care interventions
Homelessness	Work with partners in local authority and housing associations to provide housing Ensure housing needs built into Local Strategic Partnership and Local Area Agreement	Social worker to help find housing and provide ongoing support
Contact with criminal justice system; prison and probation	Ensure good links between prison service and primary care, particularly around discharge	Work closely with local prison service on individual basis; get to know probation staff in community
Domestic violence	Work with all partners in locality to develop policies for support and prevention including providing education across NHS so staff are aware of presentation and possible referral options	All staff to be aware of domestic violence and what options there are for intervention, referral and counselling
Unemployment	Promote job opportunities for groups who are socially excluded and in need of additional support	Provide advice in surgery on job seeking as well as available allowances
Need for dental treatment	One of the most common problems both of the prison population and of rough sleepers is poor dentition and there is a need for dental care that is accessible Strategic approach to meet this need should be considered	Provide accessible dental care including dental hygiene

Case study 3: older people in rural areas

Increasing life expectancy is one of the challenges of the twenty-first century. More people are living longer, and this is not just an issue of greater dependency. As the population age structure changes, so too do our expectations of staying healthy. In addition, as the numbers of older people as a percentage of the population grows, social relationships change. Many carers are themselves past retirement age and with increasing numbers of women working there is less informal care available and greater need for organizations to provide care. We all recognize the benefits of older people maintaining independent living, and the challenge for health and social care services, for communities and for primary care professionals is to provide appropriate support to enable this to happen.

The World Health Organization has recognized in its Healthy Ageing Policy that ageing is a societal issue not just something affecting older people, and that the focus should be on maintaining independent and quality lives at the all stages of the lifecourse as illustrated in Fig. 5.3.

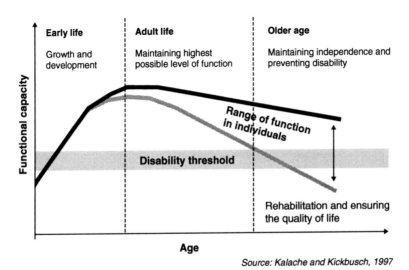

Source: Kalache and Kickbusch, 1997

Fig. 5.3 Maintaining functional capacity over the lifecourse.

The population approach of public health and the individual approach of primary care in such circumstances can be synergistic, as shown in the case study of Lucy, (See Box 5.3).

Box 5.3 Lucy

Lucy is 78. She lives in a small rural community and has managed on her own until recently, when she had a minor stroke, and walks with the aid of a stick. She is determined to carry on living in her own home, but needs a home help to get on top of the household chores. Her neighbours are very

---

Box 5.3 Lucy *(continued)*

good to her, but they go to work during the day. They do help her to get to church on Sundays and she gets visits from other churchgoers during the week. She really enjoys the lunch club which meets twice a week in the neighbouring village and relies on the local voluntary group to come and collect her. Her GP surgery is also in the next village so if her friends are busy she has to rely on a taxi to pick her up for her appointments as there is no bus through the village any more. The village shop closed 2 years ago because many of the people in Lucy's village are only there at weekends, so getting fresh fruit and vegetables can be a bit of a problem. Lucy owns her house—which is now too big for her. One of her main anxieties is that the roof is falling into disrepair—and she does not use the central heating because of the cost. Last year she slipped on the ice and broke her wrist so she tends to stay in during the winter, which can be a bit depressing.

Some of the population and individual challenges for old people such as Lucy are summarized in Table 5.4 (see p. 139).

Lucy, along with many other older people, wishes to live in the community in her own home.

As people get older, the quality rather than quantity of their life becomes increasingly important, particularly in managing the impact of chronic diseases such as diabetes and heart disease. The voluntary sector has a key role in providing information and supporting healthy living. A visit to the Age Concern website www.ageconcern.org.uk provides fact sheets on a list of ways to stay healthy: Gentle exercise; walking groups; health checks; arts projects; line dancing; and life-long learning including IT skills. All of these are important for the mental and physical health and well-being of individuals, and their inclusion is not surprising. However, the website also provides access to information on topics which might at first glance not be thought of as a health issues but which are relevant from a public health point of view. These include income; heating; crime prevention; housing; leisure and learning; volunteering 50+; intergenerational networks; ageing well, and computers and the Internet.

Keeping active is particularly important in protecting against falls, which are a major cause of disability and the leading cause of mortality in older people aged over 75 in the UK (see Box 5.4). Every year, more than 400,000 older people in England attend A&E departments following an accident and up to 14,000 people a year die in the UK as a result of an osteoporotic hip fracture[12]. Osteoporosis increases the risk of fracture when an older person falls. One in three women and one in 12 men over 50 in the UK are affected by osteoporosis, and

---

Box 5.4 Physical activity: the benefits

- Stamina or endurance—the ability to sustain activity
- Strength
- Suppleness
- Skill (e.g. learning balance and coordination, etc.)
- Improved circulation
- Mental and physical well-being
- Improved self-esteem
- Weight control
- Bone density

---

almost half of all women experience an osteoporotic fracture by the time they reach the age of 70. A fall can precipitate admission to long-term care, and fear of falling can significantly limit daily activities. Falls in later life are also a common symptom of previously unidentified health problems. Key interventions are laid out in the older peoples NSF which gives standards for public health strategies to reduce the incidence of falls in the population, guidance on treatment of osteoporosis and guidelines for community-focused care.

Why does housing matter?

Lucy's story also raises the issues about poor quality housing. Poor quality housing contains a range of features which are harmful to health—damp, mould, poor indoor air quality, higher risk of injury and fires. The relationship between poor housing and poor health is a vicious circle:

- Poor housing and ill health are associated with poverty and low income
- Ill health reduces earning ability
- One-third of disabled adults below pensionable age are in paid employment
- Around three-quarters of a million physically disabled people in Britain are inadequately housed.

Addressing housing is a key element to reducing health inequalities at all ages. For example, poor housing is linked to areas of poor access to services, lack of safe play areas for children, lack of spaces for older people to walk safely and a poor social infrastructure.

There are a series of health conditions made worse by low housing standards:

- **Cold:** decreased resistance to respiratory infection, heart disease, hypothermia

- **Damp and mould**: asthma, eczema, respiratory problems
- **Indoor pollutants and infestation**: asthma
- **Overcrowding**: increased risk of infection, emotional problems, poorer educational attainment in children, social relationship problems
- **Poor quality housing**: reduced mental well-being, falls, injuries, noise-related ill health
- **Damp**: depression in women.

Fuel poverty

Associated with poor housing are the risks to older people of fuel poverty. A household in fuel poverty is one in which >10 per cent of its income is spent on all fuel use including heating the home. Over 50 per cent of those in fuel poverty are older people, many living alone in their own house—and there are more than 2.5 million households currently in fuel poverty. In the UK, every winter there are an estimated 40,000 cold-related deaths—half are from cardio-vascular and circulatory diseases including strokes and heart attacks and one-third from respiratory disease. It is estimated that for every degree Centigrade below the winter average, there are 8000 extra deaths. This is higher than in many other colder countries. Some factors which might be relevant include colder temperatures in UK houses, including the habit of sleeping in cold unheated bedrooms. Also, unlike many colder countries, many older people do not dress up warmly enough in cold spells.

Cold homes are often also damp homes. Older people tend to spend longer at home and are more susceptible to these adverse conditions. The impact of being in a cold home includes increasing blood pressure and therefore risk of heart attacks and strokes in temperatures less than 12°C degrees (a fall of 1°C increases systolic blood pressure by 1.3 mmHg and diastolic blood pressure by 0.6 mmHg). Pain from arthritis increases, and this increases the risk of falls as manual dexterity and finger strength decrease with cold. Lack of central heating and free-standing heaters can also be obstacles contributing to falls. Cold homes may also mean less social contact, with a reluctance to invite people to a cold home, and social isolation can contribute to depression. Damp housing may also be associated with increased mental ill health problems.

Simple messages such as keep warm indoors through better insulation, take up and use grants for fuel; keep warm out of doors using warm layers of clothes; and keep physically active when outside, as well as take up 'flu vaccine and other preventative measures can help[13].

Table 5.4 Roles of public health and primary care in supporting the vulnerable elderly

Concerns	Population issues	Primary care issues
Lucy		
Stroke and residual disability	Stroke strategy needed which takes into account NSF standards and includes prevention and specialized stroke care	District nurse support by regular visits linked to the voluntary sector support and home help Regular checks of blood pressure Physio advice on regular exercises to keep supple and avoid falls, as well as deal with impaired daily active living capability Aspirin to prevent transient ischaemic attacks
Older person living alone	Help secure resources for lunch club	Make referrals/information about services available
Transport	Ensure access for elderly has strategic consideration at Board level and resources for alternatives found Make representation to bus company	Arrange transport via practice using volunteer drivers
Lack of available healthy food	Support development of innovative schemes, e.g. travelling vans selling fruit and vegetables at reasonable prices	Arrange Meals on Wheels with healthy options
Distant GP surgery	Pilot telemedicine scheme	Need for visits from practice on occasional basis but rely on telemedicine link between home and surgery
Fuel poverty	Play role in designing local fuel poverty action strategy and working with partners to ensure grants are taken up, health care staff are aware of where and how to refer	Raise awareness among health professionals to risks of hypothermia and health problems associated with fuel poverty and those people most vulnerable to the cold Look for signs of fuel poverty in the home and know what improvements can be made and what home energy efficiency grants/affordable warmth programmes are available and how to refer for advice on achieving a warm home and reducing fuel bill—cheaper supplier may be possible

Summary

Population and individual perspectives of public health and primary care are synergistic.

Primary care teams and organizations are registered populations and are concerned not only with access to care but also with those in the population not seeking care, e.g. through health-promoting activities.

Primary care staff have an important role to play with the population in their communities outside the provision of clinical care, e.g. through young peoples services, community projects and school-based work.

Addressing health inequalities and social disparities is not just the business of other agencies. Primary care practitioners can, through awareness and partnership working, play a key role in the core business of population health, starting with their own practice populations.

References

1. Tudor Hart J. *A New Kind of Doctor*. London: Merlin, 1988.
2. Wanless D. *Securing Good Health for the Whole Population*. Final report. London: HM Treasury/Department of Health, 2004.
3. Department of Health. *Our Health, Our Care, Our Say: A New Direction for Community Services*. Cm 6737. London: The Stationery Office, 2006.
4. Smithies J. Community development and primary healthcare. In: Drinkwater C, Kai J, ed. *Primary Care in Urban Disadvantaged Communities*. Oxford: Radcliffe Medical Press, 2004; 59–73.
5. Bridge Consortium. The Evaluation of the New Opportunities Fund Healthy Living Centre Second Annual Report, 2003. available at www.biglotteryfund.org.uk.
6. Putnam, R. *Bowling Alone*. New York: Simon and Schuster, 2000.
7. Teenage Pregnancy Unit. www.dfes.gov.uk/teenagepregnancy.
8. Swann C, Bowe K, McCormick G, Kosmin, M. *Teenage Pregnancy and Parenthood: A Review of Reviews. Evidence Briefing*. London: Health Development Agency, 2003.
9. FPA Factsheet: www.fpa.org.uk/about/info/teeagepregnancy.htm (accessed 12 May 2006).
10. Griffiths S, Thorpe A, Dumelow C. An audit of health care provision for rough sleepers. *Public Health Medicine* 2004; 5: 27–30.
11. Kalache A. Kickbusch I. A global strategy for healthy ageing. *World Health* 1997; 4: 4–5.
12. Department of Health. *National Service Framework for Older People I*. London: Department of Health, 2002.
13. Faculty of Public Health. *Fuel Poverty and Health Briefing Statement*. June 2004.

6

Public health in practice: improving services

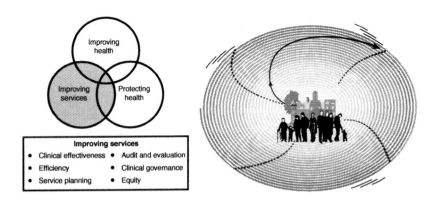

This chapter addresses the second of the three domains of public health practice, improving services.

It discusses the approaches that primary care practitioners take to improving health care for their patients and for the people in their localities, based on the hierarchy of prevention (primary, secondary and tertiary prevention) using coronary heart disease (CHD) as a case study. It also discusses screening as a specific example of secondary prevention, with the ethical dilemmas of screening a healthy population, the issue of informed consent and the role of primary care organizations (PCOs) in planning, managing, delivering and monitoring screening programmes.

The major contribution that social, economic and environmental changes have made to improving health over the last 150 years has led many to the view that health care has little effect on population health[1,2]. This view has now been challenged. For example, it is estimated that about 5 years of the 30-year increase in life expectancy in the twentieth century can be attributed to the provision of health care[3]. The most significant reason for this gain is the diagnosis and treatment of CHD, which contributes 1–2 years of these additional years of life. In addition to increasing life expectancy, health care improves quality of life, for instance in the treatment of chronic conditions such as hip replacement, cataract extraction, and drug treatment for epilepsy or diabetes. Improving health care services is therefore a central component of public health.

In Chapter 1, we discussed two models that inform public health practice. The first was the individual (high risk) versus the population (public health) approach, and the hierarchy of prevention (primary, secondary and tertiary prevention). The primary care practitioner bridges the divide between the high risk and the population approach, and provides a service to individuals and populations. This chapter will look at the primary care practitioner's role in improving the quality of health care through the application of public health knowledge and skills alongside their own clinical knowledge and skills. Because the scope of health care is so vast, we have chosen to focus in this chapter on one condition, coronary heart disease (CHD), to exemplify the role of primary care and public health teams in primary prevention (health promotion/disease prevention), secondary prevention (evidence-based treatment) and tertiary prevention (care and support in the community). It draws on the National Service Framework (NSF) for CHD[4] and other policy documents.

Delivering and improving health care

Coronary heart disease as a priority

CHD is the biggest single cause of death in the UK and a huge burden in terms of ill health, societal and health care costs. Tackling CHD prevention and treatment has been a national priority since 1992 when the government of the day published the 'Health of the Nation'[5]. It has continued to be a major priority in 'Our Healthier Nation'[6] and 'Choosing Health'[7].

CHD is a preventable disease that kills more than 110,000 people in England every year. More than 1.4 million people suffer from angina and 27,000 people have a heart attack annually. It accounts for about 3 per cent of all hospital admissions in England[8].

CHD is one of the major contributors to health inequalities in this country. Among unskilled men, the death rate is almost three times higher than it is among professionals. These differences have more than doubled in the past 20 years. For people born in the Indian subcontinent, the death rate from heart disease is 38 per cent higher for men and 43 per cent higher for women than rates for the country as a whole[8].

We use the three levels of prevention that we discussed in Chapter 1 as the framework for this Chapter (see Box 1.7). Each level has a service delivery element, we illustrate the contribution of primary prevention services with smoking cessation; of secondary prevention services with management of hypertension; and of tertiary prevention with heart failure management.

Primary prevention

This section explores the provisions of smoking cessation services as an example of primary prevention and also illustrates a needs assessment as part of the public health process.

Primary prevention aims to prevent the onset of disease by reducing factors in the population through changes in behaviour and lifestyle, supported by appropriate public policies and health education. Primary prevention is an important responsibility of primary care staff, and is remunerated as such. When new patients enrol with a practice, the practice usually offers them a health check, and a key part of that health check is to establish the patient's smoking status, and other aspects of lifestyle such as drinking and physical activity.

Why Stop Smoking Services are a priority

Smoking is the biggest single cause of illness in this country, and the Department of Health introduced a six-point action plan to tackle smoking:

- Helping smokers to give up
- Second-hand smoke
- Education and media
- Reducing tobacco promotion
- Labelling and regulation
- Taxation and smuggling.

All PCTs are required to have tobacco control strategies based on the six-point action plan, with smoking cessation services as a central part of this. Smoking Kills (1998)[9] provided a framework and funding for setting up smoking cessation services across the country and set targets for year on year improvements in smoking cessation.

The Health Development Agency (HDA) summarized the evidence base for the reduction of smoking[10] and NICE has produced guidance on brief interventions and referral for smoking cessation in primary care[11]. Advice from a GP routinely given to all patients who smoke results in about 40 per cent attempting to quit; and that intensive behavioural support plus nicotine replacement therapy or bupropion (Zyban) significantly increases an individual's chances of success.

NHS Stop Smoking Services are an important element of the Government's strategy for tackling smoking. The target is 800,000 quitters at 4 weeks between 2003 and 2006. The Department of Health recommends a multi-tiered approach to providing support as the best possible way to reach more smokers, and to gain the greatest reduction in smoking prevalence[9]. These are brief opportunistic advice to stop; intermediate interventions (one to one support); and specialist group support. These services are delivered by primary care teams or through dedicated primary care Stop Smoking Services delivered by PCOs or by the independent sector. Next we look at smoking cessation in terms of the public health process set out in Chapter 3.

Assessing the need for smoking cessation service

Table 6.1 sets out what a needs assessment for Stop Smoking Services might look like.

The size of the problem Public health specialists can establish smoking rates across the district and at smaller population levels, e.g. practices or wards.

Table 6.1 Needs assessment for smoking cessation: what would this look like?

	At PCO /LA level	At practice level
The size of the problem	Data on smoking rates from local lifestyle surveys or from synthetic estimates of smoking, by different population groups and geographical areas	Data from the practice register on smoking rates Practice staff's local knowledge of different communities and of public places such as pubs or clubs where there are high rates of smoking
What helps the problem?	Research evidence on the effectiveness and cost effectivenss of smoking cessation services[9,10]	Views of patients on what would help them
The services currently available	A review of the services available to the practice population The national helpline	A review of existing services in the PCT area, both within and outside the NHS Practice staff views on current services or lack of services Patient views on existing services

Accurate smoking data are difficult to obtain. Very few areas have up to date lifestyle survey data. So-called synthetic estimates of the data are the best available and are derived by applying the national rates obtained from national surveys such as the Health Survey for England to the local population, allowing for differences in age, sex, socio-economic condition and ethnicity. For smoking, synthetic estimates at ward level are available on the Neighbourhood Statistics site (see Chapter 4).

Practice level data tend to underestimate smoking rates. Recording is not comprehensive as remuneration is currently associated with recording for people with risk factors for heart disease or with established heart disease, and some patients rarely attend so will not have their smoking status recorded.

What helps the problem? The answer to this question relies on what the evidence tells us. The CHD national service framework[4] and the HDA review[10] on smoking cessation services provide the evidence of effectiveness and cost effectiveness from research on which to base provision of services. There would be no expectation on either PCT or practice staff to undertake reviews of the literature as this is better done nationally.

The services currently available The third element of the needs assessment requires information provided by the PCO and local practice. This is obtained from various sources, e.g. surveys of practice staff, local knowledge about other non-NHS providers, data from PCO commissioning and finance departments. Finally, a needs assessment summarizes the findings from different sources and makes recommendations for changes in services. This is used to inform the next stage, the health improvement strategy.

Planning to meet health needs

Having agreed what needs to be done, the PCO prepares a local smoking cessation strategy on the basis of the needs assessment. This is undertaken by the public health staff (Director of Public Health, tobacco control lead and CHD lead) supported by other PCO staff and by a steering group which should include practice staff and users of the service. It sets out the PCOs plans for providing smoking cessation services, what the service will involve, the availability of medication, how the service will be targeted at populations with high levels of smoking, the costs of the service, and local guidelines which set the evidence into the local context of service delivery. The strategy has targets and standards in order to assess its success.

The strategy is consulted on with key stakeholders and will be approved by the clinical executive and the PCO board before being implemented.

Smoking cessation services are delivered by practice staff and by dedicated smoking cessation services. The service delivered by practice staff will require support in terms of educational support to staff to help patients stop smoking. We talk about tools and techniques for behaviour change in patients in Chapter 4 and describe the Stages of Change model. This model was devised for people with addictions and is the model applied for smoking cessation. Practices also need to know about dedicated services so the PCO will inform all practices about the availability and referral details of local services.

Reviewing to assess impact

The service is evaluated against the targets and standards set out in the strategy. The data are collected by practices and by the local smoking cessation services according to a protocol agreed in advance, as part of the strategy. Currently the target in England is the 4 week quit rate. Smoking cessation services currently target only a small percentage of all smokers in a local area.

Some of the population and individual challenges for people like Sanjay (Box 6.1) who are at risk of heart disease are summarized in Table 6.2.

Box 6.1 Sanjay

Sanjay is in his early 50s. His parents came to Britain in the 1950s and set up a local convenience store in South London. Sanjay now manages the shop and also runs a small taxi business. He is overweight and a heavy smoker. He was recently diagnosed as a type 2 diabetic. He is having chest pain on climbing stairs. His GP has just referred him to the local hospital and he is on the waiting list for a CABG. The GP has advised Sanjay to stop smoking but he is finding it difficult.

Table 6.2 Roles of public health and primary care in preventing heart disease

Sanjay	Population issues/ public health programmes	Individual issues/primary care interventions
Smoking	Design and monitor impact of smoking cessation services	Assess individual's level of dependence and motivation to stop. Provide smoking cessation support with nicotine replacement therapy if appropriate
	Support implementation of smoke-free NHS premises and smoke-free public places	Refer to the local Stop Smoking Service

Table 6.2 (continued) Roles of public health and primary care in preventing heart disease

Sanjay	Population issues/ public health programmes	Individual issues/primary care interventions
Obesity	Work with local authority and other partners in the PCO to develop policy on healthy diets and promote physical activity	Provide advice tailored to his lifestyle Exercise prescription, referral to local walking group where available
	Use media opportunities to promote the message of healthy eating and physical activity	
Coronary heart disease (CHD)	Develop and lead implementation of local strategy for CHD based on the CHD NSF[4]	Make early diagnosis and appropriate referral to hospital; undertake ongoing management; ensure cardiac rehabilitation referral and advice
	Do a health equity audit of access to cardiac revascularization procedures.	
Diabetes	Develop and lead implementation of local strategy for diabetes based on the Diabetes NSF[12]	Education in prevention and self-management.
	Set up a diabetic retinopathy screening service	Set up nurse-led diabetes clinic in the practice, with regular disease monitoring, support and advice
		Refer for diabetic retinopathy screening

Secondary prevention

This section explores hypertension control as an example of secondary prevention and also illustrates the development and implementation of a health improvement strategy as part of the public health process. Secondary prevention aims to halt the progress of an established disease through early diagnosis and treatment, health education and treatment. (We discuss screening programmes as a special example of secondary prevention at the end of this chapter with particular reference to cardiovascular risk screening and informed choice.)

Why the management of hypertension is a priority

Hypertension is a major risk factor for stroke, CHD and other illnesses such as kidney disease and aortic aneurysm. The risk of heart disease is directly related to blood pressure: each 20 point increase in systolic blood pressure, or 10 point increase in diastolic blood pressure, doubles the risk of death from heart disease. The World Health Report 2002[13] estimated that 11 per cent of the overall disease burden in developed countries is due to high blood pressure, and that it contributes to over half of all cases of CHD.

Around 40 per cent of men, and 35 per cent of women are known to have high blood pressure. Effective treatment is available, but many people have undiagnosed or inadequately treated hypertension[8].

Hypertension is included in one of the key targets within the NHS Planning and Priorities Framework, and a NICE guideline for the management of hypertension in primary care was published in August 2004[14].

Drug treatment is recommended for blood pressure >160/100 mmHg or >140/90 mmHg for patients with raised cardiovascular risk[14]. Lifestyle changes are also effective; these include weight loss, increasing physical activity and reducing salt and alcohol intake. Blood pressure control is particularly important—and effective in reducing circulatory disease—in those with diabetes.

In the Health Survey for England, someone is regarded as having high blood pressure if their systolic pressure is ≥140 mmHg, or their diastolic pressure is ≥90 mmHg, or if they are on antihypertensive drugs. Blood pressure—and the prevalence of high blood pressure—increases with age. There is a clear social class gradient in women, with people in lower socio-economic classes having higher prevalence of high blood pressure. There is less of a social gradient in men. Many people with hypertension (around 80 per cent of men and 70 per cent of women) are not being treated, and 60 per cent of those who are receiving treatment still have high blood pressure—both worrying statistics given the contribution of high blood pressure to heart disease and stroke. Several ethnic minority groups have a lower prevalence of treated hypertension than the general population, although the overall prevalence of hypertension is higher in Pakistani and Black Caribbean women.

Assessing the need for hypertension services

What would a needs assessment for hypertension services look like (Table 6.3)?

As above, the recommendations of the needs assessment informs the next stage which is the health improvement strategy.

Table 6.3 An example of a needs assessment for hypertension services

	At PCO level	At practice level
The size of the problem	Health Survey for England, estimates at local level Data from the Quality and Outcomes Framework	Data from the practice register about patients with hypertension, and on hypertensive treatment

Table 6.3 *(continued)* An example of a needs assessment for hypertension services

	At PCO level	At practice level
What helps the problem	Research evidence on the effectiveness and cost effectivenss of hypertension treatment (this will include medication and lifestyle changes)	Views of patients on what would help them
The services currently available	A review of existing services in the PCT area, both within and outside the NHS	A review of the services available to the practice population Practice staff views on current services or lack of services Patient views on existing services

Planning to meet needs

The PCO prepares a local hypertension strategy on the basis of the needs assessment. This is undertaken by the public health staff (Director of Public Health, and CHD lead) supported by other PCO staff and by a steering group which will include practice staff. This will set out the PCOs plans for providing hypertension services, what the service will involve, how the service will be targeted at populations at higher risk such as people with diabetes, the costs of the service, and local guidelines which set the evidence into the local context of service delivery. The strategy will set targets and standards against which to assess success. Table 6.4 concentrates on secondary prevention (detecting and controlling hypertension).

Detection and control of hypertension are delivered by primary care staff. Practices have to adapt their processes and systems to improve their service to people with hypertension. The PCT should support this change with the help of

Table 6.4 Key elements of a hypertension strategy (adapted from 'Easing the Pressure: Tackling Hypertension'[15])

Where are we now?	The case for a local hypertension strategy is derived from the needs assessment and should include: • the key policy drivers—both national and local • an estimate of the local burden of hypertension • an estimate of the potential benefits of local action • a review of current activity and identification of gaps.
Where do we want to be?	Aims and objectives set the 'direction of travel' of the strategy. Standards, targets and milestones are more specific operational goals against which the whole strategy and its component strands can be evaluated. (See Table 6.5 for the practice targets through the new GMS contract.)

(Continued)

Table 6.4 *(continued)* Key elements of a hypertension strategy (adapted from 'Easing the Pressure: Tackling Hypertension'[15])

How do we involve patients and the public?	The views of patients are sought through the needs assessment. Patients should also be included in the steering group.
How do we engage/ communicate with partners?	This requires a 'whole-systems' approach, involving a range of partners in planning the strategy, steering its implementation and ensuring that it is integrated with related parallel strategies and policies. Try to build on existing partnerships, e.g. a National Service Framework implementation programme or a management programme for long-term conditions.
How can we make change happen?	**Agree local guidelines** in the context of national guidelines for detecting and managing hypertension. Guidelines emphasize the importance of assessing cardiovascular risk as a basis for prioritizing patients for antihypertensive treatment. **Prepare an implementation plan** which establishes clinical leadership, identifies facilitators to visit practices, sets up local meetings, and education and training, puts in place an audit system with feedback, produces patient information and assesses the budgetary implications. Get approval from the Professional Executive Committee and the PCT.
How do we know we have done what we wanted to do?	The two basic rules for successful evaluation are: • The evaluation process must be developed at the start, at the same time as aims, objectives and targets of the intervention are worked out. • Adequate funding must be set aside for the evaluation. A good guide is 10 per cent of a programme's budget. A clinical audit programme and a health equity audit programme need to be put in place to help improve service within practices.
How do we make successful change become normal practice?	Often funding for an initiative like this is short term. It is essential to ensure ongoing funding. This is made easier at present due to the fact that there is a big emphasis on reducing risk of heart disease and stroke. Quality payments for GPs are reflecting this (see Table 6.5).

facilitators, education and training, and support with data collection and audit. The practice staff have to work with patients to ensure concordance with treatment, and will be supported in this (see Chapter 4).

Through the new GMS contract, practices are funded to reach certain targets for hypertension detection and management. The indicators are set out in Table 6.5.

Reviewing to assess impact

The services will be evaluated against the targets and standards set out in the strategy. The data are collected by practices according to a protocol agreed in advance, as part of the strategy.

Table 6.5 Clinical indicators for hypertension from the new GMS contract

Indicator	Points[a]	Payment stages[b]
BP1. The practice can produce a register of patients with established hypertension	6	
BP4. The percentage of patients with hypertension in whom there is a record of the blood pressure in the previous 9 months	20	40–90 per cent
BP5. The percentage of patients with hypertension in whom the last blood pressure (measured in the pervious 9 months) is 150/90 mm Hg or less	57	40–70 per cent

[a]This is out of 1050 available through the Quality and Outcomes Framework.

[b]This sets out the thresholds between which a sliding scale of payment is made.

Tertiary prevention

This section explores services to manage heart failure as an example of tertiary prevention and also illustrates monitoring and evaluation as part of the public health process.

Tertiary prevention aims to prevent disease progression and attendant suffering after a disease is clinically obvious and a diagnosis established. It involves treatment, counselling and health education. We use heart failure as an example of tertiary prevention. By detecting and managing heart failure, patients' quality of life and life expectancy can be improved.

What is the rationale for investigating and managing heart failure?

Most cases of heart failure result from CHD and about a third result from hypertensive heart disease. The incidence of heart failure is about one new case per 1000 population per year. This increases with age to more than 10 cases per 1000 population in those aged 85 and over. The median age of clinical presentation is 76 years. The male to female ratio is about two to one. Population prevalence rates have been estimated as between three and 20 people per 1000, increasing to at least 80 cases per 1000 among people aged 75 and over.

Heart failure often has a poor prognosis. Despite grading heart failure by severity of symptoms, it is difficult to specify a prognosis for people with heart failure as they have a high risk of sudden death. There are thought to be about 6000 deaths a year due to heart failure associated with CHD. Annual mortality for those with heart failure ranges from 10 per cent to more than 50 per cent depending on severity. There is evidence that people with heart failure have a worse quality of life than people with most other common medical conditions. Psychosocial function is impaired, with over a third experiencing severe and prolonged depressive illness.

Heart failure accounts for about 5 per cent of all medical admissions to hospital, and people with heart failure are frequently readmitted to hospital. Indeed, readmission rates for heart failure are among the highest for any common condition in the UK and have been estimated to be as high as 50 per cent over 3 months. About half of these admissions may be preventable.

Assessing the need for heart failure services

Table 6.6 shows what a needs assessment for heart failure services would look like.

Table 6.6 Assessing health needs: sources of information at PCO and practice level

	At PCO level	At practice level
The size of the problem	Data from the Quality and Outcomes Framework Data from Hospital Episode Statistics Extrapolation of data from surveys to the PCT population	Data from the practice register about patients with heart failure, and on heart failure treatment
What helps the problem?	Research evidence on the effectiveness and cost effectivenss of heart failure treatment from NICE reviews and guidance	Views of patients on what would help them
The services currently available	A review of existing services in the PCT area, both within and outside the NHS, for diagnosis and management of heart failure.	A review of the services available to the practice population Practice staff views on current services or lack of sevices Patient views on existing services

Planning to meet needs

In heart failure, the major issues are for the PCO and primary care teams to agree and put in place models of care[16] to:

 ◆ Identify people at high risk of heart failure (e.g. people who have had a heart attack)

 ◆ Assess and investigate people with suspected heart failure

 ◆ Provide and document the delivery of appropriate advice and treatment

 ◆ Offer regular review to people with established heart failure.

Heart failure care should be delivered by a multidisciplinary team working with other health and social care worker in integrated way.

The management of heart failure is shared between health care professionals in both primary and secondary care, with patients and their carers increasingly involved in shared decision making on management. The NICE guidance[17] notes that, as with many other conditions, patient focus groups suggest that the major failings of management relate to poor communication between health care professionals, and between patients and the professionals caring for them. An important element of the strategy and implementation is improving communications between patients and their health care staff (see Chapter 4 on communicating with patients).

Services are delivered through the following routes[16]:

- Through primary care consultations in routine general practice surgeries, with the care determined by practice protocols/guidelines and appropriate forms to collect patient information.

- By 'outreach' follow-up by specialist nurses and others of people admitted to hospital with heart failure to provide education and support begun before discharge from hospital.

- By 'multidisciplinary support in the community' for those with established heart failure including home-based interventions with access to social care, the local palliative care team for ongoing support and palliative care advice as needed.

- By 'heart failure clinics' for investigation and/or follow-up. These could be located in primary care at PCO level or secondary care depending on the local circumstances. They could be successfully led by nurse practitioners or by doctors depending on local circumstances

Reviewing to assess impact

Evaluation and audit require money and time, which needs to be built into the plans for the heart failure service.

Table 6.7 sets out the indicators for each practice through the Quality and Outcomes Framework.

As well as an indication of how each practice is doing through the Quality and Outcomes Framework, a clinical audit programme needs to be put in place to ensure that practices can identify how they are performing and how they can improve services. In addition, the public health department needs to undertake a health equity audit to ensure that at the level of both practice and PCO the programme is helping to reduce inequalities through targeting for example black and minority ethnic groups.

Clinical audit (Chapter 4) is the systematic assessment of the quality of care and is an essential component of modern high quality health care and an important component of clinical governance. All primary care practitioners and practices are expected to participate in clinical audit. In addition to the

Table 6.7 Clinical indicators for heart failure from the new GMS contract 2006/07

Indicator	Points[a]	Payment stages[b]
Records HF1. The practice can produce a register of patients with heart failure Initial diagnosis	4	
HF2. The percentage of patients with a diagnosis of heart failure (diagnosed after 1 April 2006) which has been confirmed by an echocardiogram or by specialist assessment	6	40–90 per cent
On-going management HF3. The percentage of patients with a current diagnosis of heart failure due to left ventricular dysfunction who are currently treated with an angiotensin-converting enzyme inhibitor or angiotensin receptor blocker, who can tolerate therapy and for whom there is no contraindication	10	40–80 per cent

[a]This is out of 1000 available through the Quality and Outcomes Framework.
[b]This sets out the thresholds between which a sliding scale of payment is made.

indicators above, the NSF suggests the following data should be collected to measure quality improvement in primary care[16]. These are indicators not measures of access or quality.

1. Number and percentage of the registered population with a diagnosis of heart failure

2. Number and percentage of people with confirmed heart failure or left ventricular dysfunction currently prescribed an angiotensin-converting enzyme (ACE) inhibitor

3. Number and percentage of patients with a diagnosis of heart failure who have ever undergone echocardiography by practice and PCT

4. Age–sex-standardized admission rates for heart failure by PCT and Health Authority

5. Age–sex-standardized mortality rates for people with heart failure/left ventricular dysfunction

6. Number and percentage of people with heart failure for whom specialist palliative care advice has been sought by practice and PCT.

Box 6.2 gives an example of a health equity audit of primary care management of patients with heart failure, and demonstrates how data collected in primary care give a population perspective across the area.

Box 6.2 Health equity audit of heart failure management in primary care.

An inner city PCT undertook a health equity audit of heart failure in primary care. The public health team estimated the number of people living with heart failure by applying national prevalence rates to the local population. The numbers of patients with heart failure recorded at GP practices was lower than expected, whereas the hospital admission rate for heart failure was one of the highest in the country. Most of the patients with heart failure were admitted via A&E.

A review of several practice registers found that there was under-reporting of heart failure, in particular amongst ethnic minority groups.

The PCT decided to initiate a programme to improve diagnosis and management of heart failure in primary care. This involved the appointment of a heart failure specialist nurse and a GP with a special interest in cardiology. The nurse worked with GPs and nursing staff to improve knowledge about heart failure; to support the identification and management of people with heart failure; to improve recording on the GPs' clinical system; to improve the organization of care in the practices; and to ensure early referral for echocardiography. A GP with a special interest in cardiology set up and ran a clinic to see and manage the onward referral to secondary care, with the support of local cardiologists.

The audit was repeated after 2 years. The number of patients with heart failure recorded at practices had increased by 50 per cent and the increase was bigger in ethnic minority groups. The number of patients admitted to hospital had reduced by 10 per cent. The percentage of patients admitted via A&E had dropped by 20 per cent.

Screening programmes in the NHS

All screening programmes do harm, some do good as well
UK National Screening Programme.

We single out screening in a separate section as it has unique characteristics in terms of secondary prevention, offering a service to a healthy population not seeking diagnosis or care. Screening for disease before it causes clinical symptoms is intuitively appealing as it can be argued that it prevents established disease, and reduces the cost of treatment. However, screening can do harm as well as benefit, and the risks, costs and benefits to individuals and to the health service of introducing a screening test need to be taken into account.

Screening is one of the most important preventive medical activities. It can be defined as a specific, rapid examination applied to all or a specified part of the population to identify the likelihood of existing illness at a pre-symptomatic stage, or to identify susceptibility to a particular disease. At the first stage, it is not intended to be diagnostic. Screening can be 'systematic' when applied to the whole, or specific parts of the population (including systems for call and recall), or 'opportunistic' when applied to those who seek medical attention for another, perhaps unrelated condition. In practice, much screening activity in the community blends features of both approaches.

Screening in primary care

Screening activities are undertaken from primary care at all stages of the life cycle (Table 6.8). Different members of the primary care team may be involved in screening activities and to different degrees. For example, at one extreme, only administrative staff may be involved in providing home addresses for patient on a practice list to those organizing systematic breast screening programmes. At the other extreme, risk factor screening for cardiovascular disease may be initiated, undertaken and acted upon entirely in primary care. All screening activities carry an implicit ethical imperative to support

---

Box 6.3 Screening system

Screening involves a system not just a test. The following needs to be in place to deliver a service[18]

- A register for issuing invitations and reminders
- A system for checking that follow-up steps happen
- Screening tests
- Investigations
- Interventions
- Information and support for participants
- Staff training
- Policymaking
- Coordination locally and nationally
- Setting standards and ensuring they are met
- Commissioning research to improve screening.

informed choice. That is to say, patients need to understand the implications of positive findings and how they may be expected to act on them.

The proportion of time devoted to such activities in primary care will continue to increase as evidence accrues to support new screening programmes, e.g. for bowel cancer.

Table 6.8 Screening activities in primary care

Antenatal	e.g. possible haemoglobinopathies
Postnatal	e.g. for metabolic disorders such as phenylketonuria or hypothyroidism
Intrauterine	e.g. ultrasonic detection of growth retardation or anatomical defects
Childhood	e.g. periodic child health surveillance for delayed development of vision, hearing, language and cognition
Pregnancy	e.g. for anaemia, immunity to rubella
Interuterine	e.g. ultrasonic detection of growth retardation or anatomical defects
Adulthood	e.g. for cardiovascular risk factors, urinalysis for diabetes, chronic renal disease, cervical cancer
Old age	e.g. for disabilities, cognitive decline

Informing patient choice in screening

Although screening programmes may benefit populations, not all participants will benefit and some will be harmed by participation. For example, categorizing individuals as belonging to high risk groups is associated with the adverse effects resulting from labelling. The identification of diabetes, hypertension or hyperlipidaemia creates demands for clinical monitoring and adherence to drug treatment, potentially resulting in a life lived in fear of a heart attack or stroke. Many people do not want to pay these prices for an uncertain reduction in personal risk[19].

A policy shift is occurring in the UK and elsewhere towards informed choice, encouraged by the National Screening Committee[20].

An informed choice or decision has two core characteristics: first, it is based on relevant, good quality information; and, secondly, the resulting choice reflects the decision maker's values. The net effect of any population-based preventive strategy depends on the number of people participating, their baseline levels of risk and the changes in risk achieved by their actions after testing. A policy of informed choice could, in theory, increase inequalities in outcomes by increasing anxiety and avoidance in people aware of their increased risk. On the other hand, although a policy of informed choice may reduce the likelihood of the public health objectives of screening being achieved, it should increase the effectiveness of interventions among people who choose to participate and may prove at least as cost effective as current efforts[21]. A policy of informed choice places primary care back in partnership with patients seeking help to change their behaviour,

Box 6.4 Screening for coronary heart disease risk

The NSF for CHD recommends that all patients with a 10-year absolute risk of a coronary event (non-fatal myocardial infarction or death from CHD) of >30 per cent should 'be targeted and treated'[4]. People meeting or exceeding this threshold may be viewed as 'screen positive'. If such patients take effective drugs for hypercholesterolaemia and high blood pressure, they can, as a group, reduce this risk by about 30 per cent over 10 years (estimated from studies over 5 years). This might reduce a 10-year risk of 30 per cent to one of 21 per cent. Thus a patient identified as being at high risk by the screening criteria in the NSF has about a 9 per cent chance of benefiting (and a 91 per cent chance of not benefiting) from 10 years of treatment. To put this another way, 11 patients at high risk must be treated for 10 years to avoid a coronary event in one of them.

as opposed to being faced with a responsibility for improving the health of the public, regardless of the motivation of individuals.

Who's who in CHD management in public health and primary care?

Each PCT has the prevention and management of CHD as one of its top priorities, and every PCT has a CHD strategy for the whole CHD care pathway. The contributions that public health and primary care teams make to each of the steps 5 to 8 in the public health helix is set out in Table 6.9.

Box 6.5 What is a GP with a special interest in CHD[22]

(See also Chapter 8 on the primary care and public health workforce.) This has both a strategic and implementation role, the main purpose of which is to develop and streamline services for patients with CHD within the PCT in collaboration with secondary and tertiary care colleagues within the CHD networks. Locally this is the Local Network of Cardiac Care (LNCC). Additionally, the post-holder will oversee quality assurance issues in collaboration with the clinical governance lead.

The Department of Health and the Royal College of General Practitioners are developing a competency framework for GPs with a special interest, which is likely to have different competency levels with equivalency to the competency frameworks in the NHS's Agenda for Change.

Table 6.9 The public health helix: who is involved in the process from the public health and primary care teams

	Public health staff	Primary care staff
Step 5. Assessing health need At PCT level	CHD lead for PCT (usually a public health consultant or specialist) Public health information analysts	GPs (PEC chair, clinical governance lead, GP with special interest in CHD, see Box 6.5) Specialist nurse
Step 5. Assessing health need At practice level	Public health consultant Public health information analysts	GPs, community nurses and health visitors Clinical governance leads
Step 6. Planning to meet need	CHD lead (usually a public health consultant or specialist) Public health pharmacist Public health nurse	GPs (PEC chair, clinical governance lead, GP with special interest in CHD) Community pharmacist lead Community or specialist nurse lead
Step 7. Acting to address need		All members of the primary care teams including community pharmacists Social and home care staff
Step 8. Reviewing to assess impact	CHD lead (usually a public health consultant or specialist) Public health information analysts	Clinical governance lead Clinical governance team GP with a special interest Specialist nurse

Summary

This chapter looks at the complementary and interlinked roles primary care and public health practitioners have to improve the quality of health care. It is in this domain of improving health care that the two disciplines work closest. We look at the approaches using the concept of the prevention hierarchy which shows how even tertiary prevention (the diagnosis and management of people with established disease) requires the collaborative working of the two disciplines, and has an important public health impact. People working in primary care have as their major focus the health care needs of their patients, and public health approaches are central to that focus.

References

1. Illich I. *Limits to Medicine. Medical Nemesis—the Expropriation of Health*. London: Marion Boyars, 1976.
2. McKeown T. *The Role of Medicine—Dream, Mirage or Nemesis*. London: Nuffield Provincial Hospitals Trust, 1976.

3. Bunker JP. Medicine matters after all. *Journal of the Royal College of Physicians of London* 1995; 29: 105–112.

4. Department of Health. *National Service Framework for Coronary Heart Disease*. London: Department of Health, 2000.

5. Department of Health. *The Health of the Nation: A Strategy for Health in England*. London: HMSO, 1992.

6. Department of Health. *Our Healthier Nation. A Contract for Health*. Cm 3852. London: The Stationery Office, 1998.

7. Department of Health. *Choosing Health: Making Healthy Choices Easier*. Cm 6374. London: The Stationery Office, 2004.

8. Crowther R, Rolfe L, Hill A, Morgan S, Rutter H, Watson J. *Indications of Public Health in the English Regions 3: Lifestyle and its Impact on Health*. Stockton on Tees: Association of Public Health Observatories, 2004.

9. HM Government. *Smoking Kills. A White Paper on Tobacco*. London: The Stationery Office, 1998.

10. Health Development Agency. *Evidence Briefing. Smoking and Public Health: A Review of Reviews*. London: Health Development Agency, 2004.

11. National Institute for Health and Clinical Excellence. *Brief Interventions and Referral for Smoking Cessation in Primary Care and Other Settings*. Public Health Intervention Guidance 1. London, NICE, 2006.

12. Department of Health. *National Service Framework for Diabetes. Delivery Strategy*. London: Department of Health, 2002.

13. World Health Organization. *The World Health Report 2002: Reducing Risks, Promoting Healthy Life*. Geneva: World Health Organization, 2002.

14. National Institute for Clinical Excellence. *Management of Hypertension in Adults in Primary Care*. London: National Institute for Clinical Excellence; 2004.

15. Maryon-Davis A, Press V. *Easing the Pressure: Tackling Hypertension. A Toolkit for Developing a Local Strategy to Tackle High Blood Pressure*. London: Faculty of Public Health and the National Heart Forum. 2005.

16. Department of Health. *Heart Failure. National Service Framework—Coronary Heart Disease*. London: Department of Health, 2000.

17. National Institute for Clinical Excellence. *Chronic Heart Failure. Management of Chronic Heart Failure in Adults in Primary and Secondary Care*. London: National Institute for Clinical Excellence, 2003.

18. Raffle A, Barratt A, Gray M. Assuring screening programs. In: Pencheon D, Melzer D, Gray M, Guest C, ed. *Oxford Handbook of Public Health Practice*, 2nd edn. Oxford: Oxford University Press, 2006; 258–265.

19. Misselbrook D, Armstrong D. Patients' response to risk information about the benefits of treating hypertension. *British Journal of General Practice* 2001; 51:276–279.

20. National Screening Committee. *Second Report of the UK National Screening Committee*. Departments of Health for England, Scotland, Northern Ireland and Wales, 2000.

21. Marteau T, Kinmonth AL. Screening for cardiovascular risk: public health imperative or matter for individual informed choice? *British Medical Journal* 2002; 325: 78–80.

22. Department of Health. *Guidelines for the Appointment of General Practitioners with Special Interests with the Role of Service Development. Primary Care Coronary Heart Disease Lead*. London, Department of Health, 2002.

7

Public health in practice: protecting health

Jeremy Hawker and Gillian Smith

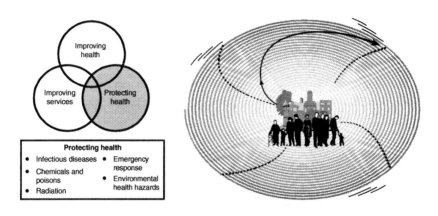

This chapter addresses the third of the three domains of public health practice, protecting health. It gives a general description of health protection issues and implications for primary care. It describes how we monitor illness associated with infections and other hazards and provides examples of prevention work for health protection. It gives examples of how primary care agencies respond to individual cases of infection and to adverse health incidents

Health protection is the third of the domains of public health practice. It is the branch of public health that deals with the control of disease related to infectious and environmental hazards. In the UK, this is generally taken to mean[1]:

- ◆ All aspects of the prevention and control of communicable disease
- ◆ Public health aspects of chemical, environmental and radiation hazards
- ◆ Health emergency planning and response to disasters.

Why is health protection important?

Health protection is an important area for public health action because:

- ◆ Many exposures to, or consequences of, infectious hazards can be reduced by preventive action by the individuals at risk
- ◆ Many other exposures to communicable and environmental hazards are outside the control of the individual at risk and require action at a community level.

Although the incidence of many infections declined in previous centuries with improved nutrition, sanitation, vaccines and developments in antimicrobials, new problems have emerged, and the burden of illness from communicable and environmental hazards is substantial. New infections (e.g. SARS, avian 'flu, HIV/AIDS) have emerged and illness as a result of environmental hazards is increasingly recognized.

Many infections do not come to the attention of health services; it is estimated that in a year, one in five individuals will suffer from an intestinal infectious disease, yet only 3 per cent will consult a GP. The cost of treating infectious disease in England has been estimated as being £6 billion each year, with primary care bearing the highest burden of the costs (£3.5 billion). It has been estimated that 40 per cent of the population consult their GP in a year because of an infection-related problem, 50 per cent of all consultations in children are for infections and 80 per cent of antibiotics are prescribed in general practice.

The contribution of environmental pollution to overall ill health is not yet accurately resolved, but global estimates conservatively attribute 8–9 per cent of the total burden of disease to it. In addition to the overall burden, illnesses from exposure to communicable and environmental hazards are perhaps the most inequitably distributed of all diseases (see later).

Although some health protection issues affect individuals and only have implications for those individuals, health protection hazards often involve more people. Table 7.1 gives examples of the potential impact on the wider population.

Several national action plans (e.g. Tuberculosis Action Plan[2], Sexual Health Strategy[3], Hepatitis C Action Plan[4]) focus on health protection issues and emphasize the importance of a multiagency approach in order to tackle issues effectively. For example, sexually transmitted infections (STIs) require diagnosis in primary care, good and accessible genitourinary services with good contact tracing, and surveillance to identify the amount and distribution of infections.

Table 7.1 Examples of how health protection issues may affect more than the individual

Health protection issue	Wider impact
Gonorrhoea, chlamydia, tuberculosis	Contact tracing conducted to screen for disease in close contacts
Meningococcal disease, unimmunized high risk contacts of influenza, pregnant non-immune contacts of chickenpox	Antimicrobial and/or immunization prophylaxis may be needed to protect others
Reported cases of food poisoning, chemical spillage, cases of avian 'flu	Need to conduct wider public health investigation/follow-up population 'at risk' and organize appropriate interventions

Surveillance in primary care

Surveillance for communicable disease and environmental hazards is essential for rapid public health action, both prevention and treatment. A description of surveillance is given in Chapter 4 including the essential contribution of data generated within primary care arising from the clinical encounter. Certain infectious diseases are notifiable by law, and these are set out Table 7.2.

Health inequalities and health protection

Health inequalities are particularly marked in infectious and environmental diseases. Relevant factors include:

♦ Socio-economic group: deaths, hospital admissions and primary care attendances for the most common gastrointestinal, respiratory and genitourinary infections are all more common in less affluent populations. Many environmental inequalities are also evident by socio-economic group, e.g. 42 per cent of children in England living within 1 km of a regulated industrial process are from the most deprived quintile of the population, compared with 7 per cent from the most affluent quintile.

♦ Ethnic group: in England, those of Black African ethnicity are 60 times more likely to have HIV infection and 90 times more likely to have TB than the white population; those of South Asian ethnicity are 40 times more likely to have TB; rates of gonorrhoea and chlamydia are 10 times higher in Black Caribbeans; serious imported infections, such as malaria, typhoid and paratyphoid are much more common in South Asians.

♦ Sexual orientation: men who have sex with men have a much higher prevalence of HIV infection and incidence of gonorrhoea and syphilis.

Table 7.2 Reporting of notifiable diseases and other infections. Confirmed or suspected cases of the following should be reported to the local CCDC. Infections marked in *italics* should be reported on the same day by telephone.

Statutorily notifiable diseases	Other infections that need to be reported for public health reasons
Anthrax	*Avian influenza*
Cholera	Campylobacter
Diphtheria	*Botulism*
Dysentery (amoebic + bacillary)	CJD
Encephalitis	Clostridium difficile
Food poisoning	Cryptosporidium
Leprosy	*E. coli O157*
Leptospirosis	Giardia
Malaria	*Legionnaires' disease*
Meningitis	Listeria
Measles	Lyme disease
Meningococcal septicaemia	MRSA
Mumps	*Psittacosis*
Ophthalmia neonatorum	Q fever
Paratyphoid fever	Salmonella
Plague	*SARS*
Poliomyelitis	
Rabies	
Relapsing fever	
Rubella	
Scarlet fever	
Smallpox	
Tetanus	
Tuberculosis (all)	
Typhoid fever	
Typhus	
Viral haemorrhagic fever	
Viral hepatitis (A/B/C/d/E)	
Whooping cough	
Yellow fever	

- Socially excluded groups: intravenous drug users have substantially increased risk of blood-borne viruses and serious systemic infections; travelling families have increased risk of vaccine-preventable diseases; refugees are at increased risks of many serious infections; prisoners are at increased risk of blood-borne viruses, hepatitis A and TB; the homeless are at increased risk of diseases related to poor living conditions such as hepatitis A; sex workers are at increased risks of STIs.

♦ Geographical inequalities are evident for many environmental hazards: e.g. less than 5 per cent of children in the South West live within 1 km of a regulated industrial process compare with 15 per cent in the North West.

Many of those inequalities, particularly in relation to ethnicity, sexual orientation and social exclusion, are of a much greater order of magnitude than those seen for non-communicable/environmental disease. In addition, many individuals may be in more than one higher risk group, e.g. the prisoner, drug user and homeless groups will overlap, and it is in the nature of most infectious diseases to spread mainly within population subgroups (people mix most with other people like them). The service implications of these inequalities is mentioned later.

Primary prevention in health protection

We describe the hierarchy of prevention in Chapter 1. Its application is as relevant in health protection as it is in the other domains of public health practice. Prevention activities aim to influence personal behaviour through the provision of advice and supporting services.

Immunization

Immunization against infectious disease has been spectacularly successful and is the most effective of specific health protection initiatives. Effective immunization services require the coordination of the inputs of many different professionals and agencies. Each local health organization, e.g. PCTs in England, should delegate a particular person (or persons) to take on special responsibility for implementing improvements to immunization programmes at local level. This person is known as the Immunization Coordinator.

The theoretical aim of immunization services is to achieve herd immunity against those diseases transmitted from person to person (e.g. measles) and to protect everyone against those with other sources (e.g. tetanus). Many countries have set general targets for immunization uptake based on the WHO approach. In the UK, these are:

♦ 95 per cent uptake of all primary immunizations, including measles, mumps and rubella (MMR), by the child's second birthday.

♦ 70 per cent uptake of annual influenza immunization in those aged over 65.

Many PCTs fail to achieve these targets. These tend to be in areas with the highest population density and therefore where a higher than average uptake is needed to achieve herd immunity. Many PCTs also vaccinate a significant proportion of their children much later than the target age: this further increases the pool of susceptibles, allowing transmission to continue. A further consequence of late vaccination is the exposure of infants to pertussis and *Haemophilus influenzae* b (Hib) at an age at which the severity of the disease is highest.

Contributing reasons for low or late immunizations are:

♦ Reduced public confidence in certain vaccines after media scares, e.g. MMR and pertussis. Concern may be highest in higher social class parents.

♦ Confusion amongst health professionals about safety and real contraindications of vaccines, particularly pertussis.

♦ Factors related to social deprivation, particularly high population mobility, lone parenthood and large family size.

♦ Factors relating to religion, lifestyle and ethnicity. Immigrant children are often not up to date with vaccination.

♦ Problems with the way programmes are organized, delivered and remunerated.

The immunization schedule in the UK was revised in 2006 (Table 7.3). These changes include the introduction of a vaccine against the seven most common strains of *Streptococcus pneumoniae* ('pneumococcus') that has already been shown to be highly effective in the USA. An estimated 50 children under 2 die each year from invasive meningococcal disease, mostly from meningitis, and up to 50 per cent of the survivors of pneumococcal meningitis have serious sequelae such as deafness, cerebral palsy and blindness.

Table 7.3 New UK immunization schedule, 2006[5]

Age	Vaccine
Neonates	BCG (high risk groups only)
	Hepatitis B (high risk groups only)
2 months	Diphtheria/tetanus/pertussis/polio/Hib (DTaP/IPV/Hib)
	Pneumococcal conjugate vaccine (PCV)
3 months	DTaP/IPV/Hib
	Meningococcus C (Men C)
4 months	DTaP/IPV/Hib
	Pneumococcal conjugate vaccine
	Men C
12 months	Hib/Men C

Table 7.3 *(continued)* New UK immunization schedule, 2006[5]

Age	Vaccine
13 months	Measles/mumps/rubella (MMRI)
	Pneumococcal conjugate vaccine
3–5 years	1 dose booster of:
	Diphtheria/tetanus/pertussis/polio (DTaP/IPV)
	Measles/mumps/rubella (MMRII)
13–18 years	1 dose of booster of:
	Diphtheria (low dose)/tetanus/polio (Td/IPV)
Adult	Boosters for tetanus and polio if appropriate
	Vaccines for occupational or lifestyle risks
65 years	Influenza
	Pneumococcus (polysaccharide vaccine)
Any age	Influenza
	Pneumococcus (medical risk groups)
	Travel vaccines

Infection control

Primary health care settings

Good infection control practices are essential in all health care settings including primary care (every practice needs to have documented procedures and protocols, e.g. for sterilization of instruments). Patients with underlying conditions making them more vulnerable to infection are increasingly being cared for in the community. Similarly, patients attending health care premises may themselves be infectious.

The importance of proper hand-washing as a cornerstone of infection control in the practice (or any health care) setting cannot be overstated. As for all health care settings, staff with gastroenteritis should not return to work until free of symptoms because of the risks of transmission of infection.

Advice on good infection control practices, e.g. cleaning, disinfection and sterilization of equipment, can be obtained from PCT Infection Control Nurses. Most PCTs will have up to date guidance on infection control in the practice settings. There should be clear policies on immunization (e.g. hepatitis B immunization) for staff and the action to be taken following a needlestick injury.

Standard measures to limit the spread of infection are given in Box 7.1.

Box 7.1 Standard precautions to limit the spread of infections[6]

- ♦ Hand hygiene: handwash with soap and water or use of an alcohol hand rub or gel. Cover wounds or skin lesions with a waterproof dressing.
- ♦ Use personal protective equipment: disposable gloves and aprons, and eye protection.
- ♦ Handle and dispose of sharps safely.
- ♦ Dispose of contaminated waste safely.
- ♦ Manage blood and body fluids: spillages and collection and transport of specimens.
- ♦ Decontaminate equipment including cleaning, disinfection and sterilization.
- ♦ Maintain a clean clinical environment.
- ♦ Prevent occupational exposure to infection and managing sharps injuries and blood splash incidents.
- ♦ Manage linen safely.
- ♦ Place patients with infections in appropriate accommodation.
- ♦ Sterilize re-usable instruments in line with national guidance and/or use of single-use instruments.
- ♦ Minimize use of toys and play equipment and documented cleaning schedules for those that are provided.

Reproduced with permission from Hawker et al: *Communicable Disease Control Handbook*, 2nd edn.[6]

Schools

In the main, children are fit and healthy—though schools settings can pose particular risks for infections. For example *Shigella sonnei* caused particular problems with schools outbreaks in the early 1990s; mumps outbreaks occurred in secondary schools in 2004/05; and influenza-like illness can spread rapidly in boarding schools. Certain infections are more common in school-aged children though are more likely to be transmitted in household settings, e.g. head lice (head to head contact is more frequent in households).

Many of the queries on infections in school children are handled by the school nurse in collaboration with the education staff, though in an outbreak the local Health Protection Unit would be involved. Following a case of meningococcal disease in a school, the Health Protection Unit will advise the school on the public health implications and provide background materials (e.g. details of signs and symptoms, see Meningitis Trust website at end). If an outbreak were to occur (e.g. more than one case of meningococcal disease within a month), then the PCT director of public health and the local health protection unit would convene an outbreak control team to manage this in collaboration with the school.

For several infections, e.g. winter vomiting or norovirus infection, it is important that children do not return to school symptomatic as the infection is likely to spread. A number of factsheets have been produced for schools on communicable disease commissioned by the Health Development Agency and Department of Health. This is part of the 'Wired for health' project. Often local guidance has been produced on infections in schools/nurseries and would be available from the local Health Protection Unit.

Care homes

Residents of care homes may have particular infection risks: underlying chronic illnesses, increased infirmity and lowered resistance to infections, and increased potential exposure to infections spreading within care homes. In addition, increasingly residents with more complex medical needs (e.g. tube feeding, urethral catheters, surgical wounds, etc.) are being cared for in community settings. Hence the risk of infections associated with health care interventions increases.

It is important that good infection control practices are instituted (see Box 7.1) and advice on infection control for care homes can be obtained through the community infection control nurses. Implementation of effective infection control may be more difficult because of staff issues, such as high turnover, and residents issues, such as dealing with residents with mental impairment.

Certain infections, e.g. influenza, can spread rapidly in the residential setting and it is important that staff are aware of how to recognize a potential outbreak and how outbreaks should be reported (to the local Health Protection Unit). Control measures can be more difficult to implement when there is no designated medical person with responsibility for all residents.

With the introduction of age-based policies for both influenza and pneumococcal vaccines, it is important that the homes are able to ensure vaccination of residents.

Prisons

PCTs now have responsibility for prison health services. Prisoners have particular health issues, with poor vaccine uptake and high-risk behaviour that may continue whilst in prison, exacerbated by the lack of adequate prevention services (e.g. needle exchange, condoms, etc.). Such individuals will sooner or later return to the community and may revolve between the two settings.

Travel health

As we gain better control of infection within the UK and as the UK population travel to more and more exotic locations, the relative importance of imported infection continues to grow. There were more than 60 million visits abroad by UK residents in 2003. Fifty per cent of travellers to the less developed world will have a health problem associated with the trip and, although the risk to individual travellers in developed countries is smaller, the large number of such travellers make this a significant problem too. Illness most commonly results from exacerbation of pre-existing medical conditions, accidents or infections. Although the most common infections are the gastrointestinal organisms that are also present in the UK, more exotic and serious infections include malaria, HIV, hepatitis, dysentery, typhoid, Legionnaires' disease, diphtheria, cholera and rabies. Primary care services are the most important component of prevention of travel-associated illness.

Risk assessment

The risk of infection is influenced by:

- Where the traveller is going
- Living conditions
- When the traveller is going and length of stay
- What the traveller will be doing
- Pre-existing medical conditions
- Distance from medical facilities.

Individuals from ethnic minorities who were born in the UK or who have lived here for many years will be equally at risk of many infectious hazards when visiting friends or relatives in their (or their family's) country of origin: however, many such travellers do not receive adequate advice.

Advice

- Hand hygiene
- Care with food, and water
- Avoidance of mosquito and tick bites
- Safe sex, drug use and medical care: of all recently reported HIV cases in UK-born heterosexuals, nearly half acquired their infection abroad
- Avoiding animal bites
- Adequate medical insurance.

Immunization

♦ Routine vaccinations should be up to date

♦ Hepatitis A and typhoid vaccines are generally recommended for all travel outside western Europe, North America and Australasia

♦ Some vaccines are recommended for travel to certain areas or at certain times, e.g. yellow fever, meningococcus, Japanese B encephalitis and tick-borne encephalitis

♦ Some vaccines may be recommended for those undertaking certain activities, e.g. hepatitis B and rabies

♦ Post-exposure prophylaxis may be recommended, such as rabies vaccine for those exposed to potential rabies sources such as an animal bite.

Advice is available from Department of Health publications[7] and the National Travel Health Network website (see later).

Malaria prevention

In 2003, 1722 cases of malaria were imported into the UK. There were 16 deaths, the majority in people who had taken inappropriate or no chemoprophylaxis. Prevention of malaria depends upon:[8]

♦ Awareness of risk by the traveller and doctor/nurse/pharmacist

♦ Bite reduction by physical and chemical measures

♦ Chemoprophylaxis with appropriate drugs

♦ Diagnosing clinical malaria promptly in returning travellers.

Influencing personal behaviour

Gastrointestinal infection is common, and most causative organisms can be transmitted from person to person. Some such as norovirus, *Shigella* and *Escherichia coli* O157 are highly transmissible, particularly within households and institutions. The likelihood of transmission can be significantly reduced by adequate hygiene, particularly washing hands after using the toilet and before preparing food. As most people affected by gastroenteritis do not consult the health service, this preventive intervention needs to get to all members of the public before they are ill.

In 2004, there were more than 780,000 STIs (chlamydia, gonorrhoea, syphilis, herpes or warts) diagnosed in England, Wales and Northern Ireland. There are also about 53,000 people living with HIV/AIDS in the UK, of which about 27 per cent are unaware of their diagnosis. The key to prevention of STIs is the adoption of 'safer sex' practices by the general population, with particular emphasis on those groups at higher risk, such as sex workers, men who have sex with men, young people and certain ethnic minorities. These messages are delivered by a multidisciplinary workforce in a range of community settings. The Government's health strategy, 'Choosing Health', includes a national campaign particularly targeted at younger men and women which aims to ensure that they understand the real risk of unprotected sex and to persuade them of the benefits of using condoms to prevent STIs and unwanted pregnancies.

Other examples include advice and services to illicit drug users to avoid injection or to use clean equipment to minimize the risk of blood-borne HIV and hepatitis B/C.

We explored the influence on individual's behaviour and at-risk communication in Chapter 4. Primary care practitioners are in regular contact with at-risk patients and will have many opportunities therefore to help address personal behaviour change.

Avoiding antimicrobial resistance

Antimicrobial resistance is not new—since antibiotics were first invented it has been known that certain organisms can be resistant to, and some can develop resistance to, antibiotics. Yet antibiotic resistance is increasing and although we think of antimicrobial resistance as being a particular problem for hospitals, resistant organisms are no respecters of boundaries. We know that patients are discharged from hospitals with resistant organisms, and increasingly there are antimicrobial-resistant organisms emerging in community and primary care settings.

It has been estimated that 80 per cent of antimicrobial prescribing occurs in primary care settings. High levels of antibiotic resistance usage have often been linked at the population level to high levels of antimicrobial prescribing—what is not so clear is the association between prescribing in individuals and the development of subsequent antimicrobial resistance. Several recent reports highlight the importance of antimicrobial resistance and emphasize the need for appropriate antimicrobial prescribing. For some areas, implementation of advice has been relatively straightforward, e.g. to shorten length of prescribing for uncomplicated urinary tract infections to 3 days (there has been a rise in the proportion of 3-day courses compared with longer courses). For other areas, implementation can be more difficult, e.g. patients may expect an antibiotic for an upper respiratory tract infection and there can be difficulties in distinguishing likely viral from possibly bacterial infections. We know that there has been an important reduction in prescribing in primary care (particularly for upper respiratory tract infections), with antibiotic prescribing reducing by over a quarter between 1995 and 2000. The recommendations of the Standing Medical

Box 7.2 Things that primary care can do: SMAC[10] and HPA guidance

- Only prescribe an antibiotic when there is likely to be a clear clinical benefit
- Use simple generic antibiotics first
- No prescribing of antibiotics for simple coughs and colds
- No prescribing for viral sore throats
- Limit prescribing for uncomplicated cystitis to 3 days in otherwise fit women
- Avoid widespread use of topical antibiotics
- Limit prescribing of antibiotics over the telephone to exceptional cases

Advisory Committee (SMAC), who examined the issue of antimicrobial resistance in relation to medical practice, are contained in Box 7.2.

Some organisms resistant to antimicrobials, e.g. methicillin-resistant *Staphylococcus aureus* (MRSA), certain strains of *E. coli* (which produce an enzyme called extended-spectrum β-lactamase, which makes them more resistant to antibiotics and makes infections such as urinary tract infections harder to treat) are being found in both hospital and community specimens[11]. It is important to stress that for most antimicrobial-resistant organisms there are alternative therapies available. Advice on the pattern of antimicrobial resistance and the management of such resistant organisms is available from the local microbiologist. Local antibiotic policies are produced by the local microbiologists and pharmacists, and reflect knowledge of local resistance patterns for, for example, the most common causes of urinary tract infections. Such guidance is usually distributed locally to GPs. National prescribing templates have been produced and are available from the Department of Health's Specialist Advisory Committee on Antimicrobial Resistance[11].

Problems can arise when patients colonized with MRSA (or other resistant organisms) are being discharged from hospital to nursing homes, or are to be admitted to hospitals. This is often because homes have not managed patients with multiresistant organisms before and may not be familiar with the infection control precautions to be taken. Usually liaison occurs between the hospital and community infection control nurses about such cases and transfers occur 'smoothly'—though if issues arise, the infection control nurses will be able to advise[12].

Working with disadvantaged or excluded groups

Illnesses associated with infectious and environmental hazards demonstrate marked inequalities (see above). To add to this, many of these groups will have a much lower uptake of preventative interventions such as immunization and screening; indeed some will not be registered for primary care services at all. As it is in the nature of most infectious diseases to spread mainly within population subgroups, the necessity for PCOs to focus on higher risk but often difficult to reach groups is obvious if inequalities are to be reduced and infections controlled. Conversely, non-targeted interventions will most easily reach those who already have the best health (and the loudest voice) and further widen inequalities. Prevention of infections that are more common in socially excluded groups needs to be included within appropriately designed holistic health services for these groups.

Some of the population and individual challenges for those with HIV/AIDS such as Joyce (see Box 7.3) are summarized in Table 7.4.

Box 7.3 Joyce

HIV/AIDS case study

Joyce is 41 years old. She left Zimbabwe 2 years ago with her family and two sons of 8 and 11 years. Like her husband, she is working in a local factory. She has few African friends in the block of flats where she lives and misses her family in Harare. Six months ago she fell pregnant accidentally and was found through antenatal screening to be HIV positive. She is devastated. She had no inkling that she was at risk and has not told her husband. Already isolated, she does not know where to turn for help.

Table 7.4 Roles of public health and primary care in supporting those with HIV/AIDS

Concerns	Population issues/public health programmes	Individual issues/ primary care interventions
Joyce		
Lack of understanding about the prevention and management of HIV in certain at-risk population groups	Rise in recent cases of heterosexually transmitted disease associated with the influx of people from sub-Saharan Africa.	Increase awareness among health and social care professionals with appropriate training including cultural awareness

Table 7.4 *(continued)* Roles of public health and primary care in supporting those with HIV/AIDS

Concerns	Population issues/public health programmes	Individual issues/ primary care interventions
Joyce		
	Address lack of understanding about the prevention and management of HIV in certain at-risk population groups	
	Initiate community-based awareness and educational programmes	
Screening	Many women are identified through antenatal screening but encouraging uptake of HIV tests among other subgroups is difficult.	Many primary health care teams remain poorly equipped to deliver appropriate pre-test counselling and support.
		Encourage uptake of HIV tests
	Devise antenatal screening programme	Provide pre-test counselling and support where appropriate
Mother to child transmission	This can be reduced to less than 1 per cent through the appropriate use of antiretroviral drugs postnatally.	Make appropriate use of antiretroviral drugs postnatally
	Medical monitoring and follow-up is essential.	Provide good model of service, e.g. use of Locally Enhanced Service provisions of new GP contract to to develop HIV management/ screening
Cultural context	Surveys among black Africans reveal distinctive attitudes and beliefs regarding screening and the disease that need to be addressed through community-based awareness and educational programmes	Provide good model of service, e.g. use of Locally Enhanced Service provisions of new GP contract to develop HIV management/screening
	Increase awareness among health and social care professionals of voluntary organizations such as Body Positive and African HIV network which provide much needed information and support to people with HIV	Provide preventive, culturally appropriate outreach programmes

(Continued)

Table 7.4 *(continued)* Roles of public health and primary care in supporting those with HIV/AIDS

Concerns	Population issues/public health programmes	Individual issues/ primary care interventions
Joyce		
	Support links with NGOs such as Body Positive and African HIV network and provide information	
Resource implications	Need to provide preventive, culturally appropriate outreach programmes against reality that most of the HIV budget goes on costly drug combinations.	Model of service, e.g. use of Locally Enhanced Service provisions of new GP contract to develop HIV management/screening
	Ensure resource implications are taken account of in local sexual health strategy	
	Review HIV budget and redirect resources from costly drug combinations to broader approach including prevention and social support.	

Secondary prevention: response to cases and incidents

Although the preferred option in all public health is primary prevention, important preventive action has to be taken to limit further spread from existing cases. Potential interventions include screening, contact tracing, prophylaxis, provision of behavioural advice, measures to promote early diagnosis and treatment of cases, and identification and control of outbreaks and incidents.

Screening programmes

There is an in-depth section on screening as a secondary preventive activity in Chapter 6 on improving health care.

Antenatal screening

Maternal blood from all pregnant women should be checked for evidence of active infection with HIV, hepatitis B (HBV) and syphilis to allow interventions to protect the baby (and treatment for the mother and contacts). For HIV-positive mothers, measures such as antiretroviral medication and avoidance of breast feeding will reduce the risk of HIV transmission to the baby from 25 per cent to 5 per cent[13]. In the case of HBV-positive mothers, hepatitis B vaccine ± immunoglobulin is given to the baby, dependent upon the level of infectivity implied by the blood test results.

Maternal blood is also checked for antibodies to rubella to check for maternal immunity should the mother come into contact with a case of rubella, which can cause severe fetal malformations. Urine screening for urinary tract infections is also undertaken.

Chlamydia screening

Chlamydia is the most commonly reported STI in the UK, and numbers have risen steadily since the mid-1990s. The prevalence is highest in young sexually active adults, especially women aged 16–24 and men aged 18–29. As most people are asymptomatic, large proportions of cases remain undiagnosed: untreated genital chlamydial infection may have serious long-term consequences, especially in women in whom it causes pelvic inflammatory disease, ectopic pregnancy and infertility. There is evidence that active case finding for genital chlamydial infection, through targeted screening of at-risk populations, can significantly reduce morbidity and is cost effective.

'Choosing Health'[9] included the introduction of a chlamydia screening programme in England, which should be fully in place by 2008. Local management (organization, delivery and monitoring) of chlamydia screening is coordinated within geographically distinct programme areas. These programme areas are managed by a local Chlamydia Screening Steering Group, chaired by a Programme Lead.

The target population of the chlamydia screening programme is:

♦ All sexually active men and women under 25 years of age who would not normally be offered a test for chlamydia (opportunistic screening); and

♦ All sexually active men and women under 25 years of age attending genitourinary medicine (GUM) clinics or other sexual health clinic.

Additionally, the programme should cover:

♦ All partners of those found positive on screening, regardless of age.

Opportunistic screening for genital chlamydial infection will be offered at a range of settings: contraception clinics (including those run in GP surgeries); young peoples' services; gynaecology departments; antenatal services; colposcopy services; termination of pregnancy services; and general practice. Screening may also be offered to the target population at additional settings, such as universities and colleges, secondary schools, prisons, military bases and outreach events.

Public health response to individual cases of infection

Examples of the public health action taken after the identification of a case by the clinician or laboratory include the following.

Gastrointestinal infection

Although most cases of gastrointestinal infection do not present to the health service, of those who do, the large majority are dealt with in primary care, and the opportunity for re-enforcement of the importance of personal and food hygiene should not be lost. In addition, some groups are at increased risk of passing gastrointestinal infection on to contacts outside the household, some of whom may be at risk of developing serious disease[14]. These groups, who should be advised to remain off work, school or nursery until well for 48 hours, are:

◆ Food handlers

◆ Health care workers

◆ Children under 5 years of age

◆ Individuals who are unable to implement good standards of hygiene.

Other infections for which exclusion from school/work plays a part in their public health management are given in Table 7.5[6].

Sexually transmitted infections

Although safer sex is key to control of STIs, early diagnosis, treatment (to render non-infectious) and contact tracing (to limit spread) are also important and are the key elements of health service interventions: hence the UK Government target on access to GUM clinics[9]. Re-enforcement of safer sex messages to such at-risk individuals is also important as re-infection is all too common. Current policy is to deliver these services more effectively by reducing barriers between primary and specialist sexual health services, involving an increased use of community services, including primary care practitioners with a special interest[9].

Tuberculosis

Over 8000 cases of TB were notified in the UK in 2005 (provisional data). Incidence rates in England have increased by about 50 per cent since the all-time low recorded in 1987 and are highest in London, followed by the conurbations of the Midlands, Yorkshire and Lancashire. About 70 per cent of cases are in ethnic minority groups (especially if born abroad), with rates highest in Black Africans, followed by south Asians. The Department of Health recently launched an action plan to combat TB[2], and NICE guidelines have been issued for prevention and treatment[15]. In addition to prevention efforts, the public health response to individual cases of TB involves contact tracing to identify

Table 7.5 Exclusion periods for common infections

Infection	Risk group	Exclusion period
Athlete's foot	–	None
Chickenpox	School/nursery; health care workers	5 days from onset of rash
Diarrhoea/vomiting (including *Campylobacter*, *Salmonella*, norovirus)	School/nursery; food handlers; health care workers; groups with poor hygiene	48 hours from last episode of loose stool or vomit
E. coli O157	All	Advice from CCDC
Glandular fever	–	None
Hand, foot and mouth	–	None
Head lice	–	None
Hepatitis A	Nursery; groups with poor hygiene; food handlers; health care workers	7 days after onset of jaundice
HBV/HCV/HIV	Health care workers	Worker to discuss with occupational health
Influenza	School/nursery	Until well enough
Influenza	Health care workers	5 days from onset of symptoms
Measles	School/nursery	5 days from onset of rash
MRSA	Care home	None (discuss infection control and treatment with CCDC or hospital infection control)
Mumps	School/nursery	5 days from onset of swollen glands
Ringworm	School/nursery	Until on treatment
Rubella	School/nursery; health care workers	5 days from onset of rash
Scabies	Care home; school/nursery	Until treated
Scarlet fever	School/nursery	5 days from onset of rash
Shingles	Health care workers	Discuss with infection control team/CCDC
Slapped cheek/Fifth disease (parvovirus)	School/nursery	None
Slapped cheek/Fifth disease (parvovirus)	Health care workers	Discuss with infection control team/CCDC
Typhoid/paratyphoid	All	Advice from CCDC
Warts/verrucae	–	None (cover lesion in pool/PE)
Whooping cough	School/nursery	5 days from commencing treatment

possible sources (to render non-infectious), those who may have acquired TB (for treatment), those who may have developed latent infection (for chemoprophylaxis) and non-immune contacts (for vaccination). Multidrug therapy and measures to maximize compliance are important to prevent the development of drug resistance: currently in the UK, about 7 per cent of cases show resistance to at least one drug.

Other infections

Other cases of infection that might require prophylaxis of exposed contacts include meningococcal disease (antibiotics and vaccine: see Box 7.4), Hib disease

---

Box 7.4 Public health response to a case of a meningococcal disease[16]

+ Ensure rapid admission to hospital and that pre-admission benzyl penicillin has been given. (Action: GP)

+ Arrange for prophylaxis for close contacts. The aim of close chemoprophylaxis is to eradicate the infecting strain from the network of close contacts, and thus prevent further cases among susceptible close contacts. Chemoprophylaxis should be given as soon as possible. Close contacts are defined as people who have had close prolonged contact with the case in the week before onset. Defining who is a close contact is usually done by the local Health Protecion Team, but they usually include household members, girlfriend/boyfriends, regular childminders and sometimes students in a hall of residence. Classroom, nursery and other social contacts do not need chemoprophylaxis. (Action: clinician supported by Health Protection Team)

+ Arrange for vaccination of close contacts if the infection is due to a vaccine-preventable strain. The aim of vaccination is to prevent late secondary cases. There is less urgency for vaccination, as chemoprophylaxis aims to prevent early secondary cases. Vaccine should be offered to all close contacts as defined above. (Action: GP supported by Health Protection Team)

+ Provide information about meningococcal disease to parents and educational establishments. The aim here is to improve the outcome of any secondary cases that may occur (by ensuring that cases seek medical attention quickly and that an appropriate index of suspicion is maintained) and to prevent rumours and anxiety by carefully explaining risks and actions. (Action: Health Protection Team).

(antibiotics and vaccine), pertussis (antibiotics and vaccine), hepatitis A (vaccine or immunoglobulin), hepatitis B (vaccine ± immunoglobulin), HIV (antivirals), chickenpox (immunoglobulin), diphtheria (antibiotics and vaccine) and avian 'flu (antivirals). Some potential exposures may also require interventions to protect the case, e.g. 'white powder' suspected deliberate release (antibiotics), rabies (vaccine ± immunoglobulin), diphtheria (antitoxin) and tetanus (vaccine).

Outbreak and incident management

Outbreak and incident management is an important aspect of the health protection response. Outbreaks of infection may be detected from routine surveillance of laboratory-diagnosed infections (where the organism is known, but not the source) or may come to light from reports from the public (where the exposure may be known, but not the organism) or from formal or informal syndromic surveillance (where neither is yet known). The public health response, which will be led by the Consultants in Communicable Disease Control (CCDCs) in England, working with environmental health and microbiology colleagues and others to a pre-agreed plan, usually comprises of the following steps[6]:

- Confirming that there is an outbreak, e.g. checking that it is not due to a change in ascertainment
- Confirming the diagnosis, using clinical and laboratory criteria to construct a case definition
- Implementing immediate control measures, e.g. to limit spread from cases or implicated premises
- Case-finding to allow quantification of the incident and produce a larger more representative group of cases for investigation
- Collecting basic data on the cases, using a semi-structured questionnaire
- Describing the cases by person, place and time using descriptive epidemiology
- Generating a hypothesis from the information collected, e.g. on the activities/exposures of cases
- Testing the hypothesis, often in a formal case–control or cohort study
- Implementing further control measures in the light of the findings
- Monitoring the effect to ensure that the outbreak is terminated.

Health protection teams also become involved in the investigation and management of acute chemical or radiological exposures and chronic environmental exposures, although other agencies may take the overall lead in some incidents: in the case of acute chemical incidents, this will usually be the police.

Exposures may occur via air, water, food or land, and may result from leakage, spillage, explosion, fire, inappropriate disposal or deliberate release. Chemical and radiation exposures may also contaminate casualties and carers, including their body, clothes and equipment. Casualties may need resuscitation, decontamination, antidotes, supportive treatment and/or intensive care. The situation may be sufficient to trigger the local NHS declaring it a 'Major Incident' and activating their pre-prepared plans.

Pandemic influenza

The last pandemic of influenza occurred in 1967/68 and, as the Chief Medical Officer for England states 'Most experts believe that it is not a question of whether there will be another severe influenza pandemic, but when'.[16] The increasing number of outbreaks in both wild birds and poultry of the avian strain of influenza H5N1 has been causing concern, and planning for influenza is intensifying at all levels.

The UK Health Departments' UK Influenza pandemic contingency plan[17] provides a national framework for an integrated response to an influenza pandemic. The plan provides guidance on the types of preparation and response needed by health services at the various phases of an influenza pandemic. These phases are designated by the World Health Organization (Box 7.5).

Box 7.5 Pandemic influenza

Inter-pandemic period

Phase 1: no new influenza virus subtypes detected in humans

Phase 2: no new influenza virus subtypes detected in humans, but a circulating animal influenza subtype poses substantial risks of human disease

Pandemic alert period

Phase 3: human infection with a new subtype(s) but no human-to-human spread

Phase 4: small cluster(s) with limited human-to-human transmission

Phase 5: large clusters but human-to-human spread is localized

The pandemic period

Phase 6: increased and sustained transmission in the general population

The post-pandemic period

Box 7.6 Effect of pandemic influenza in primary care[17]

- New health care contacts for influenza-like illness can be expected to exceed 1000 per 100,000 per week during the main pandemic period (the baseline is up to 30, and peak consultations during seasonal influenza in recent years have been 200–250 per 100,000 per week).

- Assuming a complication rate of 10 per cent, with half of those who experience complications consulting GP practices can expect to see between 50 and 250 new patients per 100,000 per week at the peak, with some form of complication.

The contingency plan contains estimates of the potential impact on primary care (Box 7.6) and other health services. Inevitably, until a pandemic emerges, it will not be clear which age groups will be particularly affected or the clinical severity, although pandemics of influenza have tended to cause more severe illness than seasonal influenza. The planning estimate given for the cumulative clinical attack rate is 25 per cent of the population affected over one or more waves of about 15 weeks each (the normal seasonal attack rate is 5–10 per cent). Overall case-fatality rates between 0.37% (based on the inter-pandemic and 1957 experience) and 2.5 per cent have been considered. Overall mortality varies considerably with age: at least a third of the total excess deaths may be in people under 65 years of age, compared with less than 5 per cent in inter-pandemic years.

Each PCT is required to have a designated pandemic influenza coordinator (usually the Director of Public Health) and to have developed contingency plans for a pandemic. Local plans should include the arrangements for: care of the large numbers of people potentially affected; treatment of designated groups with antivirals within 48 hours of the onset of symptoms; maintaining continuity of services with high staff absenteeism; infection control; personal protective equipment for staff; how other work is to be organized; and management of the interface between primary care and A&E departments. Interim guidance on planning and preparation has been produced for General Medical Practices including a checklist of additional requirements for infection control materials and a checklist for practices on current pandemic planning[18].

In addition to managing the influenza and any complications in patients, it is likely that, once a vaccine effective against the pandemic strain becomes available, primary care services will be involved in the administration of vaccine.

Guidance, including advice on the management of a traveller returning with avian influenza and on contacts of cases of avian influenza in birds, infection control advice is available on the Department of Health and Health Protection Agency (HPA) websites (see later).

In the event of a pandemic of influenza, clinical advice on the management of patients and antimicrobial guidance (for treatment of secondary infections) would be updated and be made available on the websites.

Environmental public health

Environmental health covers the effects of physical, biological and social factors in the environment on health and quality of life. Some of these issues, such as chemical hazards, radiation hazards and health emergencies are clearly within the brief of 'Health Protection' in the UK, whereas for other hazards it is less clear.

Health protection issues within environmental health include:

♦ Outdoor air quality, e.g. traffic fumes, industrial pollution, ozone

♦ Indoor air quality, e.g. passive smoking, allergens, chemicals

♦ Drinking water safety, e.g. lead, industrial pollution, pesticides

♦ Land or soil contamination, e.g. landfill sites, former industrial sites

♦ Ionizing radiation exposure, e.g. radon, medical sources, nuclear waste

♦ Non-ionizing radiation exposure, e.g. power lines, radio masts, mobile phones, ultraviolet rays.

There are 25 million known chemicals, of which more than 70,000 are in regular commercial use. Most of these have had no toxicological assessment and it is difficult to monitor their health effects because individual exposure is difficult to measure and disease outcomes such as cancer result from multifactorial and long-term causal pathways. However, as an example of how significant such chemicals might be, the possible health risks from outdoor air pollution include excess deaths and hospital admissions from cardiovascular disease; excess deaths and hospital admissions from exacerbation of chronic respiratory disease; an estimated 30 per cent of all acute exacerbations of childhood asthma; and increases in certain types of cancer[19]. Environmental public health will form an increasing important component of health protection in the future.

Control of environmental pollutants is usually based on a mixture of regulation, such as the Integrated Pollution Prevention and Control (IPPC) process for industrial sites and the Control of Major Accident Hazards Regulations (COMAH), and the setting of quality standards, such as the statutory standards for drinking water and non-statutory targets for air quality. In addition to Local Authorities, various national agencies are involved, including the Environment Agency, Health and Safety Executive, the Drinking Water Inspectorate and the Food Standards Agency.

Environmental issues usually arise as issues for public health organizations or PCOs because of either an obvious acute incident (e.g. a chemical fire or a chemical spillage) or local concern about the perceived risk of a chronic local exposure (e.g. a landfill site or an incinerator). Public concern may be heightened by a real or perceived increase in ill health locally, such as cancer or congenital anomalies for chronic exposures.

The public health response in acute incidents includes advice on the need for decontamination of those exposed, the need for protective equipment for staff, advice to the public (e.g. stay indoors, do not drink water), advice on the need for evacuation, advice on medical countermeasures and any long-term follow-up of those exposed. For chronic exposures, there is usually time for a more systematic epidemiological investigation, although it must be remembered that risk communication, risk perception and media handling are as important as scientific risk assessment where there is significant public concern.

Environmental health in its wider sense also includes housing, transport, food, occupational health and safety, sustainable development, urban regeneration, social inclusion, planning, energy and noise. These issues are traditionally the responsibility of Local Authorities and national government. Although not traditional areas of activity for the HPA, their influence on health suggests that they are a legitimate area for public health organizations or PCOs to work with others to improve health.

Health emergency planning

Health emergency planning prepares for any occurrence that

- presents a serious threat to the health of the community or
- causes disruption to health service provision or
- causes such large numbers of casualties as to require special arrangements by health services.

Such events can include

- Natural disasters, e.g. flooding
- Failure of essential services, e.g. petrol shortage, loss of water supply
- Major accidents, e.g. major transport accidents
- Disease pandemics e.g. influenza
- Terrorist incidents, e.g. explosions or release of biological, chemical or radiological hazards.

Dealing with emergencies involves a four-stage cycle of

- Prevention: to identify potential risks and attempt to minimize them
- Preparedness: involves the preparation of plans and training and exercises in their use
- Response: lasts as long as rapid interventions are required
- Recovery: to provide as rapid a return to normality as possible.

Health emergency planning is a multiagency activity. Its main legal framework is the Civil Contingencies Act 2004, which places certain legal responsibilities to plan and cooperate on a range of organizations, including PCT.

Organizational issues

The independent body with a particular remit for health protection is the HPA. The HPA Act 2004 sets out the functions of the agency as 'to protect the community (or any part of the community) against infectious diseases and other dangers to health'. The HPA has national, regional and local functions. The local tier of the HPA in England consists of 39 Health Protection Units (HPUs) usually covering a population of over a million residents (NB: at the time of writing, this is under review and teams are likely to get larger). The HPUs are staffed by consultants in communicable disease control (CCDCs), health protection nurses and support staff. The roles of the local teams are given in Table 7.6.

The HPA has a particular remit for health protection, though there are many agencies who work together to protect the public from adverse health events (see Box 7.7).

Table 7.6 Responsibilities of local health protection and primary care teams

Local health protection team[a]	Local primary care team
Core services	**Core services**
Setting up and maintaining surveillance systems	Advice to patients on prevention of infection, e.g. personal hygiene, food hygiene, safe sex and travel health
Analysing trends in infectious disease incidence	Early diagnosis and treatment of infectious cases or serious illness
Public health response to individual cases of infection	Reporting of cases to public health authorities
Investigation and control of outbreaks	Provision of suitable diagnostic samples
Proper Officer for public health legislation	Advice and prophylaxis to patients who are contacts of cases and others exposed to infectious or environmental hazards
Liaison with others involved in control of infectious disease	
Advice to Local Authorities, primary care staff and the public	Contribution to management of public health incidents affecting their population
Infection control advice and support to nursing and residential homes, and schools	Provision and promotion of immunization services
Investigation of environmental hazards	Promotion of and participation in screening services
Advice on commissioning services to prevent, control and treat infection	Responsible antimicrobial prescribing
Prevention and health promotion programmes	Chemical incident planning and management
Teaching and training	Infection control in GP premises
	Optional services
Optional services	Special interest services in sexual health
Immunization coordination	Special interest services for drug misusers
HIV prevention coordination	Gay-friendly services
Tuberculosis contact training	Outreach services for difficult to reach groups
Port health	Infection control in minor surgery
Wider emergency planning	Others, e.g. enhanced services

[a]This column was reproduced with permission from Hawker et al. Communicable Disease Control Handbook, 2nd edn.[6]

Box 7.7 Organizations and individuals involved in health protection[6]

The following gives examples of the ranges of agencies and professionals who work day to day on, or who may become involved in, health protection issues.

Primary health care

GPs, practice nurses, health visitors, community infection control nurses, school nurses, community pharmacists, PCT Directors of Public Health and public health staff, general dental practitioners.

Secondary care

Directors for Infection Prevention and Control

Medical Microbiologists

Hospital Infection Control Nurses

Infectious Disease Specialists

TB specialist and TB nurse advisers

Genitourinary medicine staff

Health Protection Agency

Consultants in Communicable Disease Control

Health Protection Nurses

HPA laboratories

Centre for Infections

The Centre for Radiation, Chemical and Environmental Hazards

Centre for Emergency Preparedness and Response

Local Authorities

Environmental health officers, teachers, home carer services.

Food Standards Agency
Universities and Colleges
Day Nurseries
Health and Safety Executive
The Department for Environment, Food and Rural Affairs
Water Companies

Useful websites

World Health Organization: http://www.who.int/en/

European CDC: http://europa.eu.int/comm/health/ph_overview/strategy/ ecdc/ecdc_en.htm

Department of Health (England): http://www.dh.gov.uk/

Health Protection Agency, England: http://www.hpa.org.uk/

CDSC Northern Ireland: http://www.cdscni.org.uk/

Health Protection Scotland: http://www.show.scot.nhs.uk/scieh/

NPHS Wales: http://www2.nphs.wales.nhs.uk/icds/

Local Health Protection Units (England): http://www.hpa.org.uk/lars_hpus.htm

National Poisons Information Service: http://www.hpa.org.uk/chemicals/ npis.htm

National Electronic Library of Infection: http://www.neli.co.uk/

Immunization information: www.immunisation.nhs.uk

National Travel Health Network and Centre: http://www.nathnac.org/

Antimicrobial resistance: www.dh.gov/policy and guidance/HealthandSocial CareTopics/AntimicrobialResistance/fs/en and

www.hpa.org.uk/infections/topics_az/antimicrobial_resistanc/menu.htm

Health Development Agency (Wired for Health): http://www.wiredforhealth. gov.uk/

National Meningitis Trust: www.meningitis-trust.org/

Meningitis Research Foundation: www.meningitis.org/

British Liver Trust: www.britishlivertrust.org.uk/

British Lung Foundation: www.lunguk.org.

References

1. Donaldson L. *Getting Ahead of the Curve*. London: Department of Health, 2002.
2. Chief Medical Officer. *Stopping Tuberculosis in England: An Action Plan from the Chief Medical Officer*. London: Department of Health, 2004.
3. Department of Health. *The National Strategy for Sexual Health and HIV Implementation Action Plan*. London: Department of Health, 2002.
4. Department of Health. *Hepatitis C: Action Plan for England*, London: Department of Health, 2004.
5. Department of Health. *Immunisation Against Infectious Diseases*. London: HMSO, 1996. Available at www.immunisation.nhs.uk (online version regularly updated).
6. Hawker J, Begg N, Blair I, Reintjes R, Weinberg J. *Communicable Disease Control Handbook*, 2nd edn. Oxford: Blackwell Science, 2005.

7. **Department of Health.** *Health Information for Overseas Travel.* London: The Stationery Office, 2001. Available at https://www.the-stationery-office.co.uk/doh/hinfo/index.htm.

8. **Bradley DJ, Bannister B.** Guidelines for malaria prevention in travellers from the United Kingdom for 2003. *Communicable Diseases and Public Health* 2003; 6: 180–199.

9. **Department of Health.** *Choosing Health. Making Healthier Choices Easier.* London: Department of Health, 2004.

10. **Standing Medical Advisory Committee Sub-Group on Antimicrobial Resistance.** *The Path of Least Resistance.* London: Department of Health, 1998.

11. **Specialist Advisory Committee on Antimicrobial Resistance (SACAR).** UK Template for Hospital Antimicrobial Guidelines. Available at http://www.advisorybodies.doh.gov.uk/sacar/index.htm (accessed 9 June 2006).

12. **Duckworth G, Heathcock R.** Guidelines on the control of methicillin-resistant *Staphylococcus aureus* in the community. Report of a combined working party of the British Society for Antimicrobial Chemotherapy and the Hospital Infection Society. *Journal of Hospital Infectections* 1995; 35:1–12.

13. **Department of Health.** *Reducing Mother to Baby Transmission of HIV.* Health Service Circular HSC 1999/183. London: Department of Health, 1999.

14. **Working Group of the former PHLS Advisory Committee on Gastrointestinal Infections.** Preventing person to person spread following gastrointestinal infections: guidelines for public health physicians and environmental health officers. *Communicable Diseases and Public Health* 2004; 7: 362–384.

15. **National Institute of Health and Clinical Excellence.** *Clinical Diagnosis and Management of Tuberculosis and Measures for its Prevention and Control.* London: NICE, 2006.

16. **PHLS Meningococcus Forum.** Guidelines for the public health management of meningococcal disease in the UK. *Communicable Diseases and Public Health* 2002; 5: 187–204.

17. **UK Health Departments' Influenza pandemic contingency plan** (October 2005 edition).

18. **Royal College of General Practitioners and the General Practitioners Committee of the British Medical Association.** *Pandemic Flu: Interim Guidance. Infection Control for General Medical Practices.* London: RCGP/BMA, 2006.

19. **Troop P, Endericks, T, Duarte-Davidson R.** *Health Protection in the 21st Century. Understanding the Burden of Disease; Preparing for the Future.* London: Health Proection Agency, 2005.

8

Education and workforce development

This chapter looks in more detail at the overlapping roles of the public health and primary care workforces. In both settings, roles are changing and the contribution of nurses, in particular, is expanding. Continuing structural reorganization continues to stretch capacity in public health, but new opportunities for professional development and education are explored. Public health and primary care practitioners who understand the complementary nature of their disciplines can mobilize each other's resources more effectively.

Introduction

The last 30 years have been chequered with pleas for closer cooperative working between primary care and public health[1,2]. Many of these envisaged the emergence of new hybrids. The best known of these was Julian Tudor Hart's 'community general practitioner'—'a new type of physician engaged in local participatory democracy to maximise the population's health'[3]. Why have such pleas so often gone unheeded?

At the heart of the relationship between general practice and public health is an ethical balance between individual and collective freedom[4]. For primary care practitioners, the roles of patient's advocate, mediator and population planner may overlap and conflict with one another[5]. There have always been plenty of GPs who understand the central role of primary care in tackling health inequalities. The history of primary care is studded with the contributions of activists working for public health on behalf of deprived communities[6]. Tudor Hart's pioneering work on heart disease prevention in Glyncorrwg provides a well known example[3]. Many practice teams work 'beyond the surgery door' to address determinants of their patients' health. The first president of the Royal College of General Practitioners (RCGP) is remembered for an epidemiological treatise on country practice[7].

Others remain less supportive because GPs are often untrained as health educators, with a narrow view of health promotion and limited experience of community development activities. Many primary care providers are politically antipathetic to social intervention in the guise of health promotion[8], particularly if the opportunity costs of such activities compromise their traditional caring role. Michael Fitzpatrick, for example, pleads for a form of medical practice that treats illness rather than regulating behaviour[9]. Such challenges to the 'tyranny of health' amount to retrenchment—withdrawal from a wider social role, a more restricted definition of medical practice. Patterns of behaviour are, after all, socially conditioned rather than pharmacologically determined. The challenge for the practitioner is to strike the right balance between protecting the autonomy of the individual and the health needs, inevitably politicized, of the wider community.

Following the foundation of the RCGP in 1952, the postgraduate training and professional development of British GPs became increasingly sophisticated. Paradoxically, as GPs have embraced new roles, the expertise and body of knowledge upon which has rested their claims to professional status have become less distinctive. In this respect, their experience mirrors that of public health doctors, who are now working alongside, and to some extent being replaced by, public health specialists from different disciplines.

Recently, the RCGP has re emphasised the role of GPs in public health[10]. With the increasing emphasis on chronic disease management, the engagement of primary care clinicians in both primary and secondary prevention has become increasingly important. They need new skills in the promotion of information and choice. With the Faculty of Public Health, the RCGP has looked at ways in which primary care clinicians could actively contribute to the public health agenda, e.g. effective delivery of specific NSFs, through screening programmes and advice on lifestyle factors.

If PCTs are to drive forward public health goals, they too must reinforce support among primary care workers for 'upstream' solutions. PCTs have an important role in supporting the public health agenda and helping to re-distribute resources within and between geographical areas, clinical disciplines and even practices. Primary care nurses, particularly health visitors, are often best equipped for the role. This chapter looks at how the development of public health skills across a range of primary care disciplines could further support for population health.

The public health workforce

In a review of the public health function, the Chief Medical Officer (CMO) of England described three levels of the work force[11]:

+ **Public health specialists:** consultants in public health who work at a senior strategic level to influence the health of the population, e.g. in PCTs or Strategic Health Authorities. These professionals have specialist knowledge and skills as required for certification and membership of the Faculty of Public Health.

- **Public health practitioners:** those who spend a major part of their time in preventive practice, e.g. health visitors, environmental health officers and community development workers. These people may be using research findings, public health information or health promotion skills in specific public health fields.

- **The wider workforce:** anyone with a role in health improvement and reducing inequalities, e.g. teachers, housing officers, social workers, doctors and health service managers. This category includes health advocates drawing advice from communities themselves. So-called 'health trainers' are being given skills to assist in providing to anyone who needs support, developing a healthier lifestyle[12]. Clearly, primary care practitioners including practice nurses and GPs fall into this category through their involvement in interventions ranging from school health checks to screening and mass vaccination programmes.

Various developments are blurring the boundaries between these three levels. The *Choosing Health* White Paper underlined the scale of the challenge facing the overstretched public health specialist workforce[12]. This is an increasingly multidisciplinary group working in a wide range of fields: public health intelligence, health promotion, health psychology, pharmacy, dentistry, health protection, environmental health and health economics. Primary care should provide one such specialist area of expertise in future.

On the other hand, diversification of the generalist work force is allowing doctors and nurses to develop special areas of expertise at this level. 'Practitioners with Special Interests' may, in future, focus on public health practice. The General Medical Council, Nursing & Midwifery Council and other registering bodies recognize the vital importance of public health knowledge and skills. Efforts to intensify public health input at an early stage of training should impact on this third level. New and more flexible models of training in public health are needed that take account of the complex mix of expertise required, if capacity is to be developed[13].

The changing primary health care team

The controversial World Health Report of 2000 placed the UK 18th in the WHO's ranking of different countries' health services[14]. That relative success was in part due to the strength of the primary care sector, particularly in bringing different health professionals together in community-based teams.

Changing players

Table 8.1 lists the people consistently involved. Other groups play a growing or substantial role. These include community psychiatric nurses, specialist outreach nurses (e.g. for palliative or stoma care) and clinical psychologists. There has been a dramatic increase in the number of counsellors attached to practices over the last 10 years. The potential importance of the social worker as team member is widely acknowledged. Coordination at the interface between health and social care is self-evidently important in the management of older people in particular. However, staff shortages and mutually unrealistic expectations sometimes hamper the development of close working relationships.

Changing loads

One consequence of the demographic and organizational changes described above is that the workload in primary care is widely perceived to have increased. In reality, appropriate measures of workload are difficult to define as working patterns change over time. Some burdens are lighter. For example, GPs nowadays do far fewer home visits. However, consultation rates have steadily increased and the advent of new technologies has helped shift care from hospital settings. The complexities of today's chronic disease management have increased 'decision density' in general practice.

Changing roles

The primary care team has been given a central role in coordinating many preventive services such as childhood immunization and cervical cancer screening. Technological advances, professional subspecialization, patient preferences for locally acceptable services as well as the government's desire to constrain health care spending will continue to drive much health care from secondary to primary care.

Only 8 per cent of the projected new professional resources in the NHS Plan were GPs and half of this increase was to be swallowed up in the extension of new specialist roles (often in secondary care)[15]. The advent of practitioners with special interests formalizes long-standing role diversification in general practice and will strengthen its appeal as a career choice.

Generalist care will increasingly be delivered by nurse (general) practitioners. 'Nurse-led' PMS pilots have seen nurses manage the majority of first contact care as well as provide overall leadership within the primary care team[16]. They have paved the way for new forms of primary care management as did their forebears for domiciliary and residential care management a decade ago. Over the coming years, pharmacists, social workers and others will challenge GPs' monopoly over primary care leadership.

Table 8.1 The primary care team

Title	Qualifications	Employed by	Brief description of role
GP	Medical degree, with several years of specific postgraduate training and vocational accreditation	Self-employed, salaried or 'freelance'	Provision of routine medical care and preventive activities. Referrals to others in the primary care team, and to secondary care. Director of the practice, which is a small business
Practice (treatment room) nurse	Fully registered nurse often with additional training	General practice	Works on the practice premises alongside the doctors. Does a variety of diagnostic and treatment procedures, e.g. screening, health promotion, minor illness and chronic disease management
Health care assistant (HCA)	Training often practice-based	General practice	Varied roles—undertaking registration checks, phlebotomy, ECGs, etc.
District nurse (DN)	Fully registered nurse with additional training	Local PCT	Has his or her own case management, but is also 'attached' to practice(s) and liases with them. May have specialist skills in incontinence, falls, ulcer management, etc.
Health visitor (HV)	Fully registered nurse with several levels of additional training	Local PCT	Position similar to DN, but works more in the field of prevention, health promotion and public health

(Continued)

Table 8.1 (*Continued*) The primary care team

Title	Qualifications	Employed by	Brief description of role
Midwife	As DN and HV with specific training in midwifery	Local PCT	Entirely responsible for their own caseload of pregnant women, but liase with general practice
Practice manager	Traditionally worked up from reception, nowadays has management training	General practice	Development and implementation of strategic plans, operational responsibilities for staffing, premises, finance and IT
Receptionist	May have no formal training although most have now attended local courses	General practice	Reception and administrative responsibilities (e.g. filing). Should not undertake medical tasks but may go on to train as HCAs
Medical secretary	May have some specific training in medical work in addition to basic secretarial training	General practice	Preparation of correspondence, other tasks, e.g. referrals audits
Pharmacist	Graduate level education and further training	Self-employed/local health authority	Local ('community') pharmacists are variably involved with general practice. Some health centres house their own pharmacists to provide general advice to groups of practices

Nursing in public health and primary care

The development of community nursing continued apace following the legislation referred to in Chapter 1. Working out of local authorities, the health visitor's role has always included a range of public health functions. Their responsibility for caseloads of children and young families embraces encouraging the uptake of immunization, health promotion and the identification of children at physical or emotional risk. School nurses also have a central role in the national child health promotion programme, e.g. in encouraging healthy lifestyles. 'Every Child Matters' identified five outcomes (being healthy, staying safe, enjoying and achieving, making a positive contribution and enjoying economic well-being) that are required for children and young people to make a positive transition into adulthood[17]. Nurses, midwives and health visitors are seen as essential collaborators in improving outcomes for the most vulnerable. Nurses make up the greater part of the NHS workforce and key challenges define their public health role (see Box 8.1)[18]. In contrast, the contribution of district nursing teams remains underdeveloped. They are ideally placed to adopt broader population-based responsibilities and have engaged, for example, in falls prevention projects. Furthermore, they could integrate health promotion work in the community with secondary prevention undertaken by nurses in the hospital sector.

The Family Doctors Charter of 1966 marked an important watershed in the evolution of primary care nursing. GPs were provided with financial incentives to employ nurses in support of their teams. Over the next 15 years, the numbers of practice nurses increased 10-fold. The latest GP contract has further encouraged the growth of nurse practitioners managing minor illness and

Box 8.1 Factors central to public health nursing

- Knowing what the health needs of the population are—not just those on your caseload or waiting in surgery
- Making sure services are accessible to those whose needs are greatest
- Working with others—and not just those in the health service—to tackle the wider determinants of health
- Getting local people involved in what you do
- Being ready to respond to infectious disease outbreaks and other threats to health
- Using evidence on effective practice

chronic disease. The steady diversification of primary care nursing roles is a quiet revolution with major implications for public health practice. While the first contact and continuing care roles of practice-based nurses are quickly evolving, their potential in terms of broader health promotion remains undeveloped. In part, this reflects the financial incentives introduced under the new GP contract. Leaders are required to support these developments, not least to establish the training capacity required to 'grow' public health specialist nurses.

Role of public health in primary care organizations

Public health specialists are already thinly distributed, but the demand for their skills at all levels of the NHS and local government has increased to unprecedented levels. Successive NHS reorganizations have highlighted the need for local primary care staff with public health skills. Closer working has long been the rallying cry, but without public health leadership new training opportunities will be lost. The establishment of PCTs was supposed to provide an opportunity to move the public health function into a closer relationship with primary care and local government. The continuing evolution of primary care, and in particular the re-emergence of practice-based commissioning, once more raises these expectations.

The role of the Director of Public Health reflects 10 key areas of practice. Table 8.2 sets out the main tasks of the PCT public health specialist workforce mapped against these 10 areas[19]. Most of these functions can only be delivered in partnership with colleagues in primary care or local government. As GPs take up the reins of commissioning, the challenge for specialist public health staff is to consider how best their skills in areas such as health needs assessment, information analysis and reviewing effectiveness can support colleagues in the community. This will require greater capacity than exists at the moment, and primary care staff are well placed to develop new roles. Practitioners with a special interest in public health are needed to roll out skills across practices collaborating in primary care commissioning.

New public health teaching networks are being set up across each region that create networks of public health teachers who can pool and share resources. They should offer training opportunities for GPs, community nurses, primary care teams, pharmacists and others seeking to improve health and reduce inequalities. They will need to be mindful of a variant of the inverse prevention law whereby teams working in the neediest areas are the least well developed or able to exploit new training opportunities[20,21]. Training support may therefore need to be targeted.

Table 8.2 Ten key areas of practice for the DPH

Key area	Examples of tasks
Surveillance, assessment of population health	Lead and coordinate the assessment of health needs and inequalities, identify areas for action within the local population, establish systems for health surveillance. Monitor local basket of health inequalities indicators. Lead health equity audits and produce an annual report.
Promoting and protecting population's health and well-being	Responsibility for provision of screening programmes for the local population and meeting targets for screening and immunization/vaccination programmes. Leading PCT contribution in support of surveillance, health protection and environmental control. Develop/lead health improvement initiatives and strategies.
Developing quality and risk within an evaluative culture	Develop effective clinical governance systems. Support evidence-based practice within multiprofessional teams, the evaluation of the effectiveness of health care provision and the development of appropriate health outcome measures.
Developing health services and reducing inequalities	Establishing local targets for health improvement and the reduction of inequalities. Contributing public health leadership to the commissioning process.
Policy and strategy development and implementation	Develop local health strategy including advising on effective evidence-based health care delivery.
Strategic leadership for health	Lead the PCT's contribution to building partnerships and widening participation in the health agenda.
Working with and for communities	Take a leadership role with local communities in helping them to tackle long-standing health inequalities.
Research and development	Work with information managers in the PCT and local authority to develop the information base.
Ethically managing self, people and resources (including education and continuing professional development)	Effective leadership of the primary health team, including management and staff development

Educational opportunities

Several initiatives are designed to modernize working practice and ensure a workforce better fitted for future purpose. All health professional bodies are committed to flexible training often expressed in terms of 'the skills escalator'. This 'climbing frame' is a model for education which incorporates development of modular assessment and accreditation against explicit standards. (Fig. 8.1). The career framework demonstrates the concept of a flexible career and skills escalation, enabling staff with transferable, competency-based skills to progress their career while meeting the needs of the organization.[22] Career pathways need to be developed at all levels of practice within the NHS and beyond in discussion with professional groups, educators, registering bodies, employers and the public.

Agenda for Change, a new pay system which is creating pay comparability across different disciplines, is defining the knowledge and skills required for every job in the NHS in relation to pay progression[23].

Specific public health competencies have been developed in the areas of health improvement and public health intelligence, which have allowed the development of a specific career framework for public health practitioners. Table 8.3 shows the career framework mapped against the public health/health improvement profiles developed for the evaluation of jobs through *Agenda for Change*. The process for ensuring the skills escalator and resultant career progression is

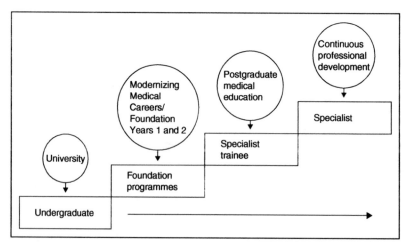

Fig. 8.1 Examples of skills escalator: medical career pathway.

Table 8.3 The career framework for health and its relationship to public health job profiles

Band		Public health job profiles
9	More senior staff	Consultant
8 a, b, c, d	Consultant practitioners	Health Improvement Principal
7	Advanced practitioners	Health Improvement Practitioner Advanced
6	Senior practitioners/specialist practitioners	Health Improvement Practitioner Specialist
5	Practitioners	Health Improvement Practitioner
4	Assistant practitioners/associate practitioners	Health Improvement Resource Assistant Higher Level
3	Senior health care assistants/technicians	Health Improvement Resource Assistant
2	Support workers	Health Improvement, Clerical Officer
1	Initial entry level jobs	

under development. The approach has, however, helped ensure equivalency across different disciplines and has clarified the competency requirements for public health. It is easy to see how primary care practitioners can move sideways into and then upwards in a public health career.

At the time of writing, adoption of *Agenda for Change* is voluntary in general practice. In future, primary care should provide a setting for one of a number of different public health roles for which competencies need to be defined. This will allow health professionals from different disciplines to identify their own extra training needs. If not too bureaucratic and cumbersome, such a framework should aid transparency and multidisciplinary working. Box 8.2 lists competencies that might be considered relevant for primary care-based public health leaders, including leadership skills. These skills are essential for effective participation in practice-based commissioning. Indeed without locally accessible public health expertise, it is difficult to see how this government initiative can succeed.

In summary, public health and primary care practitioners who understand the complementary nature of their disciplines (Table 8.4) will mobilize each other's resources more effectively.

Box 8.2 GP with special interest in public health—possible competencies

A. **Assessment of community's health needs (including interpreting information and statistics). You should be able to ...**

1. Describe the causes of the most common diseases afflicting your local population.

2. Use routinely available data to describe the health of a practice population and compare it with that of other small populations.

3. Understand the need to standardize rates of disease.

4. Demonstrate an understanding of the links between socio-economic status and health needs.

5. Assess the importance of different risk factors in a given population, including socio-economic, ethnic and genetic factors in the genesis of specific diseases or conditions.

6. Recognize inequity and discrimination and its impact on health.

B. **Promoting health, disease prevention (including screening). You should be able to ...**

1. Analyse health problems in terms of risk factors, including consideration of avoidable, relative and absolute risk.

2. Describe the features of an effective screening programme.

3. Understand the theoretical models of behaviour change and their relevance to the practice of health promotion.

4. Understand the principles involved in childhood immunization programmes.

5. Appreciate the general principles of outbreak management, and understand the role of the consultant in communicable disease control and the Health Protection Agency.

6. Describe the main causes of occupational ill health in this country and approaches to their prevention.

7. Understand the importance of addressing the wider determinants of health within communities, e.g. housing, employment and education.

C. **Setting priorities and rationing. You should be able to...**

1. Demonstrate up-to-date knowledge of the organization of the NHS.

2. Define criteria with which to guide the allocation or rationing of scarce resources.

3. Describe ethical tensions inherent in this aspect of doctors' work.

Box 8.2 GP with special interest in public health—possible competencies *(continued)*

D. Evaluating health services and clinical governance. You should be able to …

1. Demonstrate an understanding of different perspectives on the nature of 'quality' in health care.

2. Describe different ways of assessing outcomes, recognizing qualitative measures, patient acceptability and quality of life as key outcomes for health interventions.

3. Understand how the principles of evaluation, audit and standard setting help you to improve the quality of your own practice.

E. Critical appraisal skills and evidence-based medicine. You should be able to …

1. Understand the strengths and limitations of different study types and be able to appraise the quality of research critically.

2. Examine evidence of effectiveness for a specific intervention, e.g. drug, surgical procedure.

3. Turn a complex clinical or public health problem into an answerable question.

4. Conduct literature reviews to look for primary and secondary research, using electronic databases, to define a search strategy and summarize results of it.

5. Explain clinical risks in comprehensible numerical terms to patients.

F. Leadership skills. You should be able to …

1. Understand the principles of good communication.

2. Articulate strategic priorities.

3. Identify opportunities for team development.

4. Adapt to the changing external environment.

Table 8.4 Public health and primary care practitioners—core competencies contrasted

Public health practitioners	Primary care practitioners
Care for populations	**Care for individuals on practice lists**
Use of environmental, social, organizational, legislative interventions	Use of predominantly medical, technical interventions
Prevention through the organized efforts of society	Care of the sick as their prime function with the consultation as central
Application of public health sciences (e.g. epidemiology/medical statistics)	Application of broad clinical training and knowledge about local patterns of disease
Skills in health services research, report and policy writing	Skills in clinical management and communicating with individuals
Analysis of information on populations and their health in large areas	Analysis of detailed practice/disease registers and information on individuals
Use of networks that are administrative: health and social care authorities, voluntary organizations	Use of networks that are clinical rather than managerial: frontline health and social care providers, other primary care terms

References

1. **Hannay DR.** Primary care and public health: too far apart. *British Medial Journal* 1993; 307; 516–517.
2. **Ashton J.** Public health and primary care: towards a common agenda. *Public Health* 1990; 104: 387–398.
3. **Tudor Hart J.** *A New Kind of Doctor.* London: Merlin Press, 1988.
4. **Pratt J.** *Practitioners and Practices. A Conflict of Values?* Oxford: Radcliffe Medical Press, 1995.
5. **Bhopal, RJ.** Public health medicine and primary health care: convergent, divergent or parallel? *Journal of Epidemiology and Community Health* 1995; 49: 113–116.
6. **Heritage Z,** ed. *Community Participation in Primary Care.* Occasional Paper 64. Royal College of General Practitioners, 1994.
7. **Pickles W.** *Epidemiology in Country Practice.* Baltimore: Williams & Wilkins, 1939.
8. **Skrabanek P.** *The Death of Humane Medicine and the Rise of Coercive Healthism.* London: Social Affairs Unit, 1994.
9. **Fitzpatrick, M.** *The Tyranny of Health—Doctors and the Regulation of Lifestyle.* London: Routledge, 2001.
10. **Griffiths S, Haslam D.** Putting public health practice into primary care practice: practical implications of implementing the changes in shifting the balance of power in England. *Journal of Public Health Medicine* 2000; 24: 243–245.
11. **Chief Medical Officer.** *Annual Report of the Chief Medical Officer 2000.* Department of Health, London, 2000.

12. **Department of Health.** *Choosing Health: Making Healthy Choices Easier.* London: Department of Health, 2004.

13. **Griffiths S, Thorpe A, Wright J.** *Change and Development in Specialist Public Health Practice.* Oxford: Radcliffe Publishing, 2005.

14. **World Health Organization.** *Health Systems: Improving Performance.* Geneva: WHO, 2000.

15. **Department of Health.** *The NHS Plan: A Plan for Investment, a Plan for Reform.* London: HMSO, 2000.

16. **Lewis R, Gillam S, ed.** *Transforming Primary Care. Personal Medical Services in the New NHS.* London: King's Fund, 1999.

17. **Her Majesty's Treasury.** *Every Child Matters.* Cm 5860. London: The Stationery Office, 2003.

18. **Department of Health and Community Practitioners' and Health Visitors' Association.** *Liberating the Public Health Talents of Community Practitioners and Health Visitors.* London: Department of Health, 2003.

19. **Faculty of Public Health.** *Good Public Health Practice. Standards for Public Health Practice.* London: FPH, 2001.

20. **Acheson D.** *Independent Inquiry into Inequalities in Health (Acheson Report).* London: The Stationery Office, 1998.

21. **NHS Centre for Reviews and Dissemination.** *Evidence from Systematic Reviews of the Research Relevant to Implementing the 'Wider Public Health' Agenda.* York: University of York, NHS Centre for Reviews and Dissemination, 2000.

22. **Skills for Health.** *What is the Career Framework for Health?* Bristol: Skills for Health, 2005.

23. **NHS Executive.** *Agenda for Change—Modernizing the NHS Pay System.* Health Service Circular, 1999/035.

9

Epilogue

Bridging the divide—future challenges

Our intention in this book has been to explore the interaction between primary care and population health. Pleas for closer cooperative working between primary care and public health have often gone unheeded. Indeed, there are reasons for fearing their divergence with the NHS in such constant flux. In Chapter 2, we signalled concerns that conflicting policy objectives may weaken our primary care system. In Chapter 8, we examined the overstretched public health workforce's limited capacity to support colleagues in primary care. In this final chapter, we examine basic principles that need to be protected and how the two disciplines need to evolve if further progress is to be made in aligning them.

What kind of primary care?

The central importance of primary care for public health has long been acknowledged. In 1978 at Alma Ata, primary health care was declared to be the key to delivering 'Health For All' by the year 2000. Primary health care 'based on practical, scientifically sound and socially acceptable methods and technology made universally accessible through people's full participation and at a cost that the community and country can afford' was carefully distinguished from primary medical care[1]. The social and political goals of those epochal declarations—acknowledging as they did the social and economic determinants of health—were subsequently diluted. So-called 'selective primary health care' and packages of low cost interventions such as GOBI-FFF (growth monitoring, oral rehydration, breast feeding, immunization; female education, family spacing, food supplements) in some respects distorted the spirit of Alma Ata[2]. There is a fundamental difference between health care that is multisectoral, preventive, participatory and decentralized, and low cost (low quality), curative treatment aimed at the poorest and most marginalized segments of the population, particularly if that care is provided through programmes that are parallel to the rest of the health care system.

From the population perspective, a central argument for primary care is ethical: the concern with equity. Ensuring equal access to care when needed is difficult. One well-attested form of differential access to care is the so-called 'inverse prevention' effect whereby communities most at risk of ill health tend to experience the least satisfactory access to the full range of preventive services[3]. User charges for primary care have been repeatedly shown to deter those most likely to benefit from preventive activities[4].

Primary care is also often defined in terms of 'four Cs': it is continuous, comprehensive, the point of first contact and coordinates other care. This coordinating function underlines a second argument in support of primary care: the economic concern with efficiency and cost effectiveness. International comparisons of the extent to which health systems are primary care oriented suggest that those countries with more generalist family doctors with registered lists acting as gatekeepers are more likely to deliver better health outcomes, lower costs and greater public satisfaction[5]. Reviewing European primary care, Boerma has emphasized the benefits of strong primary care in developing teamwork and collaboration which helps smooth the interface with secondary care and increase patient responsiveness. In addition, screening, monitoring and follow-up can only be effectively carried out by the coordinated efforts of various professional groups on the basis of the population they serve[6].

More can be done to improve the effectiveness of primary care in delivering public health. With more clinical work shifted into the community, there is less space for preventive activities. Even those primary care practitioners who have internalized a commitment to such work find it hard when the financial environment provides no incentives for such work. The dearth of evidence in support of many preventive interventions highlights the need for further research. Reasons for the failure to implement best practice go beyond the quality of the research, and accumulating further technical evidence may not be the most useful response. Barriers to implementation include a consistent failure to address the opportunity costs of different activities in primary care. For example, increasing primary care's public health role means doing less of something else. Related to this is a failure to define adequately and with all relevant stakeholders, the public health role of primary care. This is not a technical agenda but one of achieving shared values as a starting point for any changes in professional roles.

The difficulty of transposing health systems across international boundaries is widely acknowledged. Care at the level of the community within any system reflects different histories and cultural contexts. No single model of primary health care can be universally applied[7]. Thus the principles above find variable expression in different parts of the globe. For example, in much of the Western Pacific region, the principles of equity, community involvement, intersectoral action and appropriate technology at affordable costs are promoted for primary health care systems. However, China demonstrates some of the challenges in translating the theory of best primary care practice into practice[8]. The lack of affordable health care leaves many Chinese people unable to gain access to basic primary care. Escalating costs, an ageing society, poor public health systems and weak administration are compounded by poor pay for doctors who make up their earnings by charging for medicines and diagnostic tests. People do not come forward for treatment, avoiding operations or leaving hospital early because they cannot afford to pay. As in the USA families have to make difficult decisions about how to care for their elderly relatives with limited resources, and may go into severe debt to pay medical bills.

Future developments in the UK

Developing public health practice in primary care in the UK raises different challenges. Successive reforms have attempted to consolidate a 'primary care-led' NHS. The term 'primary care' is conflated with care provided primarily through general practice under the organizational umbrella of PCTs (or their Celtic equivalents). These organizations have population responsibilities and are *de facto* public health organizations. The universal access to a GP that each citizen can expect and treatment free at the point of need can only be dreamt of in many countries. Yet the NHS is under constant review and is enduring further change.

Underpinning the apparent failure of successive models of primary care-based commissioning lies a central question. Why is the so-called shift of service provision from secondary to primary care so difficult to achieve? One part of the problem lies in the 'small business' model of general practice that has served general practice so well down the decades. The responsiveness and entrepreneurialism of 9000 practice units has adapted remarkably to successive policy directives (as targets achieved in the first year of their new General Medical Services contract have graphically illustrated). Yet, even large practices have neither the financial incentives nor the capacity to invest in surgical and diagnostic services, let alone to work proactively to address health inequalities.

At the moment, primary care is organized around small localities. The strength of this model has been the continuity of care provided by a GP serving an unchanging population in a small area over lifetimes. Increasingly, population mobility and global influences such as the Internet are blurring concepts of locality, especially in cities. Services and the people who provide them have now to contend with 'discontinuity' and how best to join up inevitably fragmented care.

There are many ways of scaling up PCOs[9]. Groups of practices operating from large primary care centres, pooling managerial resources to achieve economies of scale, could provide conventional General Medical Services alongside many services currently provided in secondary care and appropriate community-based services, e.g. pharmacy, dentistry and optometry. They might be registered companies or not-for-profit organizations, owned by GPs and other primary care professionals, and could evolve from successful practice-based commissioning collaborations. Large private companies working on an industrial model, employing GPs in networks, are moving onto the same territory. Mutuals or cooperative, not-for-profit, organizations may be more congruent with NHS' core values.

These models could facilitate the move of services away from acute hospitals and may have the potential to equip the GPs better in tackling health inequalities. Larger organizations can bring the full range of primary care services to poorer areas where currently these services are weakest. Larger populations would yield more meaningful public health data with which to target services. Specific needs such as the language requirements of minority ethnic groups could be addressed more efficiently at this level. With critical mass, such organizations could create direct links with social services and community-based voluntary organizations engaged in health promotion with specific groups.

However, this path could amount to the surreptitious privatization of the NHS. Would a mixed economy of providers be able to sustain core NHS values? There is plenty of evidence that private companies deliver costlier care that is not always more efficient or of higher quality, and may account first and foremost to their shareholders. Nevertheless, a wholly tax-funded service is increasingly difficult to sustain, and this direction of travel in policy terms is well entrenched.

What kind of public health?

The epidemiologist Geoffrey Rose famously described two broad approaches to prevention[10]. The high-risk strategy aims to protect those individuals at the high end of the risk distribution. They are usually a small proportion of that distribution. The population strategy aims to reduce the underlying causes. It is concerned with factors that affect the whole population. The high-risk strategy avoids interference with those who are not at special risk. Interventions are appropriate to the individuals targeted, and this strategy is regularly accommodated within the ethos and organization of medical care. However, the high-risk strategy has less impact on the behaviour of populations and has hitherto been limited by our ability to predict individual's futures. Population strategies, on the other hand, by tackling behaviours and other risk factors en masse, offer large benefits for populations (though the benefits to the individuals may be small—the so-called prevention paradox).

Public health specialists argue that the power resides with population strategies, but recent evidence suggests that Rose's dichotomy is less clear cut. Low to middle income countries have yet to gain from simple policy changes aimed at smoking and dietary change. However, wealthier countries able to implement strategies targeted at individuals on the basis of baseline risks will see major health benefits from medical interventions delivered via primary care[11].

The locus of public health practice is changing too. In the 1980s, public health was synonymous with restrictive management. The specialty lost its way and needed to refocus not just on health service issues but on major determinants of population health, for example working across local government. Reflecting on progress over the last 25 years, it is always possible to highlight the gaps. In most countries, population-based initiatives and quality-based frameworks have been implemented piecemeal. More can be done to make addressing health inequalities an explicit policy driver in the UK. For example, under their new contract, primary care practitioners and organizations can be reimbursed for tackling problems such as childhood obesity. On the other hand, in a world dominated by liberal, free market economies, public health and health promotion practice can be viewed as ideologically paternalistic and collectivist. Public health practitioners may be pressed to embrace approaches such as social marketing that emphasize individual rights and citizens' demands for more power in shaping state-provided services[12].

The public health approach we have emphasized brings together public health and primary care in a systematic way rooted in communities and reliant on skilled professionals. Primary care and public health are both multi-disciplinary endeavours. New cadres of primary care nurses are taking responsibility for minor illness management, triage and routine care of common chronic diseases. Public health practitioners are emerging from a range of non-medical backgrounds. Many exponents of joint working have envisaged new hybrids. A generation on, might Julian Tudor Hart's 'community general practitioner'—engaged in local participatory democracy to maximise the population's health[13]—finally emerge? WHO stresses that public health competencies, especially as they relate to the management of chronic disease, will be of increasing importance to the twenty-first century global health care workforce[14].

In conclusion, the practice of public health and primary care will continue to change and develop. Our first chapters sought to reflect the historical basis and current organizational context of public health and primary care with specific reference to England. The subsequent chapters describe approaches, the public health helix, the tools of public health and their application in the three domains of public health practice. Chapter 8 describes training which will underpin the practice. Primary care cannot stand still organizationally, and reform is inevitable as the UK faces the same pressures on its health system as the rest of the world. Nor can the public health community remain untouched by these forces. They too are challenged to make major issues such as sustainability, equity and community needs of every day relevant to primary care practitioners. The opportunities presented by the synergy of their different perspectives within a culture that focuses on health as a right, health care free when needed and a population approach that promotes prevention as well as treatment and care should not be squandered.

References

1. World Health Organization. *Primary Health Care*. Report of the International Conference on Primary Health Care, Alma Ata, USSR, 6–12 September 1978. Geneva: World Health Organization.

2. Tejada de Rivero D. Alma-Ata revisited. *Perspectives in Health* 2003; 8: 1–6.

3. Acheson D. *Independent Inquiry into Inequalities in Health (Acheson Report)*. London: The Stationery Office, 1998.

4. NHS Centre for Reviews and Dissemination. *Evidence from Systematic Reviews of the Research Relevant to Implementing the 'Wider Public Health' Agenda*. York: University of York, NHS Centre for Reviews and Dissemination, 2000.

5. Macinko J, Starfield B, Shi L. The contribution of primary care systems to health outcomes within Organization for Economic Cooperation and Development (OECD) countries, 1970–1998. *Health Services Research* 2003; 38: 831–865.

6. Boerma W. Coordination and integration in European primary care. In: Saltman R, Rico A, Boerma W, ed. *Public Health in the Driving Seat*. European Observatory on Health Systems and Policy, 2006.

7. Mullan F, Epstein L. Community-oriented primary care: new relevance in a changing world. *American Journal of Public Health* 2002; 92: 1748–1755.

8. Watts J. China's rural health reforms tackle entrenched inequalities. *Lancet* 2006; 367: 1564–1565.

9. Corrigan P. *Size Matters—Making GP Services Fit for Purpose*. New Health Network, London, 2005.

10. Rose G. *The Strategy of Preventive Medicine*. Oxford: Oxford University Press, 1992.

11. Jackson R, Lynch J, Harper S. Preventing coronary heart disease. *British Medical Journal* 2006; 332: 617–618.

12. French J. The market dominated future of public health. In: *A Reader in Promoting Public Health*. Sage/Open University, 2006 in press.

13. Tudor Hart J. *A New Kind of Doctor*. London: Merlin Press, 1988.

14. World Health Organization. *Preparing A Workforce for the 21st Century: The Challenge of Chronic Conditions*. Geneva: World Health Organization, 2005.

Index